Study Guide for

Maternal-Child Nursing Care

Mary-Ann Towle
Ellise Adams

Julie Ann Will, RN, MSN
Ivy Tech Community College of Indiana
Terre Haute, Indiana
Kim Cooper, RN, MSN
Ivy Tech Community College of Indiana
Terre Haute, Indiana
Jan Weust, RN, MSN
Ivy Tech Community College of Indiana
Terre Haute, Indiana

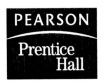

PEARSON
Prentice Hall

Upper Saddle River, New Jersey 07458

Notice: Care has been taken to confirm the accuracy of the information presented in this book. The authors, editors, and the publisher, however, cannot accept any responsibility for errors or omissions or for consequences from application of the information in this book and make no warranty, express or implied, with respect to its contents.

The authors and the publisher have exerted every effort to ensure that drug selections and dosages set forth in this text are in accord with current recommendations and practice at time of publication. However, in view of ongoing research, changes in government regulations, and the constant flow of information relating to drug therapy and drug reactions, the reader is urged to check the package inserts of all drugs for any change in indications of dosage and for added warnings and precautions. This is particularly important when the recommended agent is a new and/or infrequently employed drug.

The authors and publisher disclaim all responsibility for any liability, loss, injury, or damage incurred as a consequence, directly or indirectly, of the use and application of any of the contents of this volume.

Pearson Prentice Hall™ is a trademark of Pearson Education, Inc.
Pearson® is a registered trademark of Pearson plc
Prentice Hall® is a registered trademark of Pearson Education, Inc.

Pearson Education LTD.
Pearson Education Australia PTY, Limited
Pearson Education Singapore, Pte. Ltd
Pearson Education North Asia Ltd
Pearson Education, Canada, Ltd

Pearson Educación de Mexico, S.A. de C.V.
Pearson Education—Japan
Pearson Education Malaysia, Pte. Ltd
Pearson Education, Upper Saddle River, New Jersey

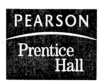

13 14 V036 15 14 13
ISBN 10:   0-13-113727-1
ISBN 13: 978-0-13-113727-1

Contents

Preface

Students entering the field of nursing have a tremendous amount to learn in a very short time. This **Study Guide for *Maternal-Child Nursing Care*** is designed to reinforce the knowledge that you-the student-has gained in each chapter and to help you master the critical concepts.

At the beginning of each chapter in this Study Guide, you will find a MediaLink box. Just as in the main textbook, this box identifies for you all the specific media resources and activities available for that chapter on the ***Prentice Hall Nursing MediaLink CD-ROM,*** found in the main textbook and the Companion Website. You will find references to animations from the **Prentice Hall Nursing MediaLink CD-ROM** and case studies and care plans from the Companion Website to help you visualize and comprehend difficult concepts. Chapter by chapter, this MediaLink box hones your critical thinking skills and enables you to apply concepts from the book.

In addition, each chapter includes a variety of questions and activities to help you comprehend difficult concepts and reinforce basic knowledge gained from textbook reading assignments. Following is a list of features included in this edition that will enhance your learning experience:

- A short introductory paragraph summarizing the objective of each chapter.
- **Matching** exercises that contain key terms and definitions from each chapter.
- Thorough assessment of essential information in the text is provided through the **Fill in the Blank** activities.
- **Multiple Choice** questions that provide you with additional review on key topics.
- **Critical Thinking Activities** that apply concepts from the textbook to real nursing scenarios.
- **Answers** are included in the Appendix to provide immediate reinforcement and to permit you to check the accuracy of your work.

It is our hope that this Study Guide will serve as a valuable learning tool and will contribute to your success in the nursing profession.

Chapter 1

The LPN/LVN in Maternal-Child, Community-Based Nursing

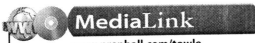

MediaLink

www.prenhall.com/towle

Use the address above to access the free, interactive Companion Website created for this textbook. Get hints, instant feedback to chapter-related NCLEX®-style questions. Link to other interesting sites.

Audio Glossary:

Use the Companion Website, or the CD-ROM disk enclosed with your textbook, to hear the pronunciation of key terms in the chapter.

Numerous health care advances have been made over the past 50 years. These changes have affected the health and wellness of the childbearing/child-rearing family as well as the nurses who provide care to them. These advances have served to reduce mortality and morbidity rates as well as made changes in the delivery of the nursing care provided.

MATCHING

Match the term in the left column with the correct definition in the right column.

1. _____ Objective data

    A. Includes the physical, psychological, and spiritual aspects of the person

2. _____ Subjective data

    B. The process of making generalized statements from a limited set of facts

3. _____ Holistic

    C. Disease prevention activities

4. _____ Nursing diagnoses

    D. Client conditions that nurses are qualified to manage independently

5. _____ Outcome

    E. Data that is measurable or can be observed

6. _____ Medical diagnoses

    F. Client goals relating to a specific nursing diagnosis

7. _____ Primary care

    G. The management of chronic, terminal, or complicated, diseases or disorders

8. _____ Secondary care

    H. Data reported from the client's personal experience/reports

9. _____ Tertiary care

    I. Statements concerning a disease process or disorder

10. _____ Inductive reasoning

    J. Activities designed to promote recovery from an acute disorder or disease process

FILL IN THE BLANKS

Fill in the blanks with the appropriate word or phrase.

1. Maternal-child nursing is care of the woman through _____, _____, and _____.

2. The Nurses Association of the American College of Obstetricians and Gynecologists (NAACOG) has been renamed the _____.

3. The medical science related to the diagnosis and treatment of childhood illnesses is known as _____.

4. Nursing actions geared toward assisting the client toward an improvement in health are known as _____.

5. _____ describes the number of deaths over a given period of time for selected population.

6. The occurrence of disease states and disorders for a specific population for a defined period of time is termed _____.

7. An experienced LPN/LVN is able to demonstrate the ability to care for clients in a culturally sensitive manner. These abilities are now second nature. This nurse is demonstrating _____.

MULTIPLE CHOICE

Circle the answer that best completes the following statements.

1. Clients who postpone childbirth for several years may face challenges. Which of the following challenges may affect the childbearing experience of the older client? Select all that apply.
   1. Increased fertility
   2. Increased risk of fetal anomalies
   3. Increased risk of Down syndrome
   4. Increased incidence of infertility

2. Until the middle of the 20th century, health care followed the medical model. This theory involved:
   1. The collaboration between the physician and the nurse.
   2. The dominance of women in nursing.
   3. The medical control of health care.
   4. Independence in nursing.

3. The greatest influence/impact on the involvement of the LPN/LVN in the care of the client is based on the:
   1. Nurse's skills and experience.
   2. State's nurse practice act.
   3. Policies of the facility where the nurse is employed.
   4. Nurse–client ratio.

4. The LPN/LVN is assisting the RN with the development of a plan of care for a pregnant client. List the order of the steps of the nursing process.
   1. Evaluation
   2. Assessment
   3. Implementation
   4. Diagnosis

5. A client assigned to the LPN/LVN requires nursing treatments permitted by the Nurse Practice Act in their state. The care interventions were not taught in the LPN/LVN's nursing education program. Using the Decision-Making Model, what is the next action the nurse should take?
   1. Ask another nurse to do the task.
   2. Perform the actions.
   3. Contact the charge nurse.
   4. Refuse to perform the treatments.

6. Which statement regarding maternal mortality in the United States is correct?
   1. Maternal mortality rates are increasing.
   2. The incidence of maternal deaths is on the decline.
   3. Studies have not identified a means to reduce maternal mortality.
   4. Prenatal care does not have an impact on maternal mortality.

7. Leading causes of infant mortality have been identified as (select all that apply):
   1. Congenital anomalies.
   2. Sudden infant death syndrome.
   3. Placental insufficiency.
   4. Low birth weight.

8. The LPN/LVN is assisting the RN to prepare a tertiary care program for clients diagnosed with osteoporosis. Which of the listed activities would best meet this criterion?
   1. A program demonstrating low-impact, low-stress exercise activities to promote and maintain mobility.
   2. A program reviewing the diagnostic tests available to screen for osteoporosis.
   3. A presentation by a dietitian focusing on the dietary prevention of osteoporosis.
   4. A video identifying clients at risk for the development of osteoporosis.

9. When considering the role of the nurse in relation to the health care team, which statement is most reflective?
   1. The nurse is the leader of the health care delivery team.
   2. The nurse's role is to carry out the treatment plan designed by the physician.
   3. Nurses are members of a multidisciplinary team.
   4. Nursing is right beneath the level of the physician.

10. A recently hired graduate PN/VN has been assigned to work closely with a preceptor. The graduate nurse has concerns about how to determine which tasks they are legally allowed to perform. What advice should the preceptor provide to the graduate?
    1. "The role of the LPN/LVN is first defined by the state's nurse practice act."
    2. "LPNs/LVNs are allowed to do everything the RN is able to do."
    3. "The hospital administration is in charge of what a LPN/LVN is legally allowed to do."
    4. "If you see another nurse performing the skill, you can do it as well."

11. The LPN/LVN is assigned to supervise a newly hired nursing assistant. When delegating tasks to the nursing assistant, what are the responsibilities of the LPN/LVN?
    1. The LPN/LVN must review the work completed by the nursing assistant.
    2. The LPN/LVN does not have any legal responsibility for the nursing assistant.
    3. The LPN/LVN will need to observe the nursing assistant to evaluate their competence.
    4. The nursing assistant is charged with the responsibility of communicating personal skill competency to the LPN/LVN.

12. Once a task has been delegated to the unlicensed assistive personnel, what is the most important responsibility of the LPN/LVN?
    1. The LPN/LVN is not responsible for delegated tasks.
    2. The LPN/LVN must document the work completed by the unlicensed assistive personnel.
    3. The LPN/LVN must provide specific directions for task completion.
    4. The LPN/LVN is responsible for assessing client receptiveness to the unlicensed personnel.

13. A student nurse is performing an assessment on the pregnant client. After the assessment, the student is preparing to document the findings. Which of the findings should be documented as objective data?
    1. Fetal heart tones are at 129, strong and regular.
    2. The client reports feelings of fatigue.
    3. The client has facial edema and complains of frequent headaches.
    4. The client is having difficulty sleeping at night.

14. The LPN/LVN is caring for a client who is hospitalized with gestational diabetes. When assisting the RN to develop the nursing care plan, the LPN/LVN and RN discuss potential client outcomes. Which of the following is most appropriate?
    1. The client will state understanding of dietary management for the condition.
    2. The nurse will teach the client dietary options for the management of the condition.
    3. The physician will prescribe a sliding scale of insulin to manage the condition.
    4. The dietitian will provide education regarding the dietary elements in the client's plan of care.

15. The LPN/LVN has noticed the policy for a procedure in the facility's manual does not appear to be current. What actions should be taken by the LPN/LVN first?
    1. The LPN/LVN is obligated to report this potential lapse to the state's board of nursing.
    2. A call to the facility's accrediting agency is indicated.
    3. The chief of the medical staff should be made aware of the concerns of the nurse.
    4. The LPN/LVN must contact their immediate supervisor regarding the concerns.

CRITICAL THINKING EXERCISE

Read the case study. Answer the questions, keeping in mind the steps of the nursing process: assessing, diagnosing, planning, implementing, and evaluating.

The LPN/LVN has been assigned to provide care to a postpartum client on the day shift. The client has been experiencing weakness in her left leg. The physician has documented that the client may be discharged if this condition resolves spontaneously. The client is having an uneventful postdelivery experience.

1. The LPN/LVN has been provided an unlicensed assistive personnel (UAP). Identify tasks the nurse may delegate to the UAP.
2. The client has requested assistance with ambulation. The LPN/LVN is providing care to another client. Can the LPN/LVN delegate this task to the UAP? Why or why not?
3. If some of the tasks delegated to the UAP cannot be completed in the time requested by the LPN/LVN, what is required?
4. The LPN/LVN has assisted the client with ambulation. Once the ambulation abilities have been assessed, what are the responsibilities of the nurse?

Chapter 2

Legal and Ethical Issues in Maternal-Child Nursing

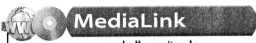

www.prenhall.com/towle

Use the address above to access the free, interactive Companion Website created for this textbook. Get hints, instant feedback to chapter-related NCLEX®-style questions. Link to other interesting sites.

Audio Glossary:

Use the Companion Website, or the CD-ROM disk enclosed with your textbook, to hear the pronunciation of key terms in the chapter.

The role of the nurse in the care of the childbearing family can be challenging. Ethical issues may arise that require the nurse to deliver quality care in the face of conflicts with personal beliefs. When these situations occur, the nurse must remain true to the profession of nursing and deliver safe, quality, nonjudgmental care.

MATCHING

Match the term in the left column with the correct definition in the right column.

1. _____ Ethics	A. Permits minors to make certain decisions concerning treatment
2. _____ Informed consent	B. Guidelines providing a framework for nursing practice
3. _____ Mature minor act	C. A written approval for treatment following a discussion of the procedure
4. _____ Confidentiality	D. A system of values and ideas that shape one's beliefs
5. _____ Ethics committees	E. A group of individuals who meet to share common concerns
6. _____ Support group	F. Maintaining the secrecy of privileged information
7. _____ Patient Bill of Rights	G. The expectations a client can expect to have met during a hospitalization
8. _____ Reportable disease	H. A group responsible for making treatment recommendations or decisions regarding complex medical issues
9. _____ State Practice Act	I. A health state presenting a public health hazard

FILL IN THE BLANKS

Fill in the blanks with the appropriate word or phrase.

1. A government-authored document discussing the opportunities for Americans to become increasingly responsible for their health care is

   _____.

2. A married 16-year-old is now able to provide consent for her own treatment because she is considered to be _____ in the eyes of the law.

3. The _____ requires health care institutions to inform clients of their rights to treatment, including advanced directives or living wills.

4. Clients experiencing difficulty conceiving a child may opt to pursue _____ to achieve a pregnancy.

5. When preparing to administer medications, a nurse must check five safety measures, which include _____ to reduce potential errors.

6. The nurse is expected to check the five Rights of Medication Administration _____ times before administering a drug.

7. A pregnant client reports lacking the financial resources to purchase adequate nutritional foods during the pregnancy. The nurse should provide a referral to _____.

8. The Patient's Bill of Rights was developed and accepted by _____.

9. An adolescent may request treatment for a _____, _____, _____, or _____ without parental notification.

MULTIPLE CHOICE

Circle the answer that best completes the following statements.

1. A nursing instructor presents an overview and discussion of *Healthy People 2000* and *Healthy People 2010* to a group of nursing students. Which of the following statements by a nursing student indicates the need for further teaching?
   1. "The American Medical Association developed *Healthy People* as a set of guidelines for physicians."
   2. "*Healthy People 2000* and *2010* encourage all Americans to take responsibility for their health care needs."
   3. "Factors that determine an individual's health are presented in *Healthy People 2000*."
   4. "*Healthy People 2000* and *2010* review the problems of the disadvantaged in having suitable access to quality health care."

2. A healthy baby boy is born to a 16-year-old client. The baby is scheduled to undergo a circumcision. Which of the following statements by the nurse to the baby's mother concerning the provision of informed consent for the procedure is most correct?
   1. "You will need to have your parents sign any consent for your baby."
   2. "Legally your parents will be in complete control of your baby's medical care."
   3. "You have the right to sign consent documents for your child."
   4. "Because you are not married, you must consult with the hospital attorney concerning the consent forms."

3. A 16-year-old client reports to the ambulatory care clinic for complaints of a backache. Bruises are found on the client's back, shoulders, and upper arms. The client's reports of how she got the bruises do not match their appearance. Which of the following actions by the nurse is most appropriate?
   1. Do nothing, as the client has provided an explanation concerning the bruises.
   2. Point out the bruises to the parents.
   3. Advise the client to contact social services if needed.
   4. Follow the facility policy for reporting suspected abuse.

4. During a routine physical examination, a female client reports she and her partner are considering treatment for infertility. The client asks the nurse for a referral to a specialist for treatment. Which of the following actions by the nurse is most appropriate?
   1. Provide the client with the name and number of a local infertility clinic.
   2. Contact an infertility clinic and obtain an appointment for the client.
   3. Do nothing, as the client must make her own contact with infertility clinics.
   4. Encourage the client to speak with the physician regarding her concerns.

5. A nurse working on the pediatrics unit must have an understanding when situations arise in which a parent or legal guardian is not allowed to make health care decisions for his or her children. Which of the following events will negate the decision-making authority of a parent or guardian?
   1. A 13-year-old child refuses to take the antibiotic whose administration the parents have approved.
   2. The nurse has consent forms for completion, and the parent appears intoxicated.
   3. The parents desire lifesaving treatments for their dying child despite the apparent futility of the situation.
   4. The parent is 17 years old.

6. A 14-year-old child is hospitalized for a urinary tract infection. During the data collection, the client asks the nurse to keep a secret about her boyfriend. Which response by the nurse is most appropriate?
   1. "Of course, I can keep what you tell me a secret."
   2. "I am not comfortable with your request."
   3. "I am legally required to report anything that may cause you harm."
   4. "You should talk to your parents about these secrets."

7. An adult client is seen in the ambulatory care clinic with manifestations consistent with a sexually transmitted infection. A specimen is collected and sent to the lab. The test results will not be available for the next 48 hours. The client tells the nurse she is embarrassed and doesn't want anyone to know about this problem. Which of following statements by the nurse is appropriate? Select all that apply.
   1. "I would not want anyone to know either."
   2. "I know just how you feel."
   3. "The diagnosis of certain sexually transmitted disorders must be reported by law."
   4. "Your diagnosis will be handled in a confidential and legal manner."

8. A recent graduate from a PN/VN program is orienting to the pediatric unit. The graduate is discussing the facility policies and legal requirements for reporting suspicions of child abuse. Which of the statements indicate the need for further teaching? Select all that apply.
   1. "I may be held legally responsible if the reports of child abuse I make do not pan out."
   2. "If my assessment identifies suspicions of child abuse, I am legally required to file a report."
   3. "If child abuse is suspected, a 'cooling off' period is recommended between the assessment and filing of the report to the proper authorities."
   4. "Failure to report suspicions of abuse may result in legal action being taken against me."

9. The parents of a 2-week-old baby ask the nurse to collect a vial of their baby's blood to put in the bank for use later. Which of the statements by the nurse is correct?
   1. "Cord blood can only be collected for banking at the time of delivery."
   2. "Have you consulted with your physician about this decision?"
   3. "Do you have approval from your insurance company to bank your baby's blood?"
   4. "You will need to determine a location to bank your baby's blood."

10. A client is injured as a result of a fall on the hospital unit. The family pursues a lawsuit against the facility. What responsibility does the practical/vocational nurse have during the litigation?
    1. The practical/vocational nurse cannot legally offer testimony.
    2. The practical/vocational nurse can relay their information to the facility's attorney for reporting.
    3. Depositions cannot be legally given by the practical/vocational nurse.
    4. The practical/vocational nurse may be required to provide documentation or testimony.

11. A client is admitted to the facility with suspicions of child abuse. After completing an assessment, the nurse selects nursing diagnoses for the plan of care. Which of the nursing diagnoses listed is of the highest priority?
    1. Deficient Knowledge Related to the Role of Social Services
    2. Altered Family Processes Related to Suspicions of Child Abuse
    3. Risk for Injury Related to Physical Abuse
    4. Anxiety Related to Hospitalization

12. A pregnant client reports her husband has recently had an affair. She states she has not made a decision about the future of her marriage. During the exchange, she asks for the nurse's opinion. Which of the statements by the nurse is most appropriate?
    1. "If it were me, I would leave him."
    2. "I don't feel comfortable sharing my views."
    3. "It will be illegal to divorce while you are pregnant."
    4. "Do you want a divorce?"

13. The LPN/LVN is assigned to provide care to a child diagnosed with renal failure. The parents advise the nurse they have decided to stop all treatments on their child. What should the nurse do first?
    1. Do nothing, as removal of treatment is within the rights of the parents.
    2. Continue to administer treatments.
    3. Contact the RN in charge.
    4. Call the hospital attorney.

14. When faced with an ethical decision, identify in order the steps the LPN/LVN must take.
    1. Identify value conflicts.
    2. Collect information.
    3. Identify the ethical issues or concerns of the situation.
    4. Define personal and professional moral positions on the issues.

15. A 15-year-old client is admitted with what is initially thought to be injuries from a "bicycle accident." During a nurse–client interaction, the teen divulges the incident was not accidental but an attempt to cause self-harm. The teen states that he has learned his lesson and will not try anything else. The teen requests the nurse maintain confidentiality and not tell anyone about the attempt. What action should be taken by the nurse?
    1. Nothing, as the nurse is bound by the rules of confidentiality.
    2. Contact the client's parents.
    3. Contact the nursing supervisor.
    4. Initiate a referral to social services.

CRITICAL THINKING EXERCISE

Read the case study. Answer the questions, keeping in mind the steps of the nursing process: assessing, diagnosing, planning, implementing, and evaluating.

A 2-year-old boy has been admitted to the pediatric care unit for observation after presenting with signs and symptoms consistent with an acute appendicitis. Diagnostic testing confirmed the diagnosis. The client's mother is a 16-year-old and unmarried. Surgery has been scheduled.

1. Who has the responsibility to discuss and provide education concerning the procedure that will be performed?
2. Given the age of the client's mother, who will be responsible for signing the consent?

3. What events may limit the ability of a parent or guardian to give consent for medical treatments for their minor child?

4. In the event the parent or guardian does not wish to have her child receive treatment, what will happen?

5. If the LPN/LVN does not agree with the plan of care desired by the client, what can the LPN/LVN do?

6. Do children have the right to refuse treatment?

Chapter 3

Nursing Care of the Family

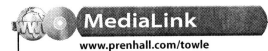

Families are the building blocks of society. Over the past several years the face of the family has changed. Despite these differences, all families are concerned with the health and wellness of their members. When providing care to families, the nurse's responsibilities involve assessment of the family type, determination of family needs, and the provision of care needed.

MATCHING

Match the term in the left column with the correct definition in the right column.

1. _____ Nuclear family
2. _____ Extended family
3. _____ Blended family
4. _____ Communal family
5. _____ Single-parent family
6. _____ Role
7. _____ Religion
8. _____ Race

A. A diagram that demonstrates relationships between family members

B. A family unit including adults and children who may or may not be related

C. A situation in which one or both spouses have children from a previous relationship

D. The traditional family consisting of parents and biological offspring

E. Belief in a superhuman power recognized as the governor or creator

F. Expectations and behaviors associated with a position within the family

G. A network of relatives and friends living within a 50-mile radius who take an active role in the emotional support of the family

H. A group of individuals who are defined by common biological deviations

9. _____ Genogram

I. Associated with the degree to which parents foster assertion and self-regulation as well as the receptiveness to demands of the children in the family

10. _____ Responsiveness

J. A family being cared for by an unmarried parent

FILL IN THE BLANKS

Fill in the blanks with the appropriate word or phrase.

1. The _____ describes the changes a family undergoes over time.

2. _____ is treatment/care designed to encompass both the client and their family system or unit.

3. Two or more people who live together and are related by marriage or blood compose a _____.

4. In a(n) _____ family, a single leader makes all decisions for the combined family groups.

5. The style of behavior, patterns, and beliefs is known as _____.

6. A nurse states she knows all African Americans act the same way. This is an example of _____.

7. When reviewing parenting styles, _____ relates to the demands parents make on children concerning expectations for mature behavior, discipline, and supervision.

8. The nurse prepares a diagram of interactions between family members and the immediate environment. The figure developed is known as a(n) _____.

9. The nurse is drawing a genomap of the family. The nurse uses _____ to identify relationships between members of the family.

10. The American Black (African American) family is frequently headed by _____.

MULTIPLE CHOICE

Circle the answer that best completes the following statements.

1. The LPN/LVN is assisting the RN to plan a teaching session with the family of a hospitalized infant in preparation for discharge. In preparation for this session, the nurse refers to the culture theory. Which of the following are concerns addressed in this theory? Select all that apply.
   1. The primary language spoken within the home.
   2. The financial capabilities of the family members.
   3. The process for decision making within the family.
   4. The number of children in the family.

2. The LPN/LVN is evaluating the performance of a nursing assistant. Which of the following statements made by the assistant would warrant further investigation?
    1. "The family does not believe in the mother working outside the home."
    2. "I am not certain about the role of the father in that family."
    3. "Those types of people will always cause trouble."
    4. "I need more information about that culture's particular beliefs."

3. Which of the following statements concerning families is correct?
    1. The number of families composed of unmarried partners is decreasing.
    2. The number of interracial families in the United States is on the rise.
    3. More than 5 million children in the United States receive care from guardians or foster care.
    4. Blended families are seldom a source of conflict.

4. During the data collection phase, a client reveals to the nurse they are a part of a communal family. Based on your knowledge, which of the following is the most correct about this family unit?
    1. The parents and grandparents live together.
    2. The children are parented by a same-sex couple.
    3. The family shares responsibilities and decisions with other families.
    4. A group leader controls the family finances.

5. According to the family systems theory, the ability of the family to manage stressors is based on:
    1. the financial stability of the family.
    2. the likelihood the family will seek assistance from outside sources.
    3. the health of the family when stressors occur.
    4. the size of the family unit.

6. The nurse has performed an assessment on a family unit. When applying the culture theory, which of the following factors should be considered? Select all that apply.
    1. Communication
    2. Space
    3. Role
    4. Size

7. A recent graduate nurse is attending a program about communication skills. After the program, the graduate nurse is discussing the session with their preceptor. Which of the statements by the graduate nurse indicates the need for further education?
    1. "Communication with families of differing backgrounds can be a challenge for the nurse."
    2. "The best way to assess a client's intent is by his or her verbal statements."
    3. "Volume of the nurse–client interaction can affect its outcome."
    4. "Some ethnic groups engage in louder interactions than other groups."

8. A client is admitted to the hospital. During the admission process, which of the actions by the nurse may be considered a violation of space by a client? Select all that apply.
   1. Putting the client's personal belongings into the closet.
   2. Sitting on the client's bed during the data collection phase.
   3. Standing during the data collection phase.
   4. Asking the client if assistance will be needed to unpack belongings.

9. A nurse is providing an educational program regarding ethnicity. As the nurse prepares the offering, which of the following components should be discussed in the determination of ethnic identity?
   1. Race
   2. Geographic location
   3. Employment history
   4. Physical attributes

10. A child is admitted to the inpatient unit. The nurse discusses the family assessment with the new graduate nurse. After the assessment, the nurse asks the graduate questions to assess understanding. Which of the statements by the graduate indicates the need for further teaching?
    1. The family assessment is an ongoing process.
    2. The family assessment examines the relationships between family members.
    3. The family assessment examines the functioning of the family.
    4. The family assessment begins with a discussion concerning the economical needs of the unit.

11. A comprehensive understanding of the family unit requires knowledge of the roles and functions of the family unit. Which of the following are primary functions of the family?
    1. Provide economic support to the family members.
    2. Offer social acceptance to members of the community.
    3. Deliver economic goods to the members of the chosen religious faith.
    4. Provide friendship to neighbors.

12. A genogram is prepared to represent a family's relationships. When reviewing the diagram, the nurse notes a double circle that is linked to a square with a broken line. Which interpretation of this is correct?
    1. The client is married to the square.
    2. The client is estranged from his sister.
    3. The client has a stepbrother.
    4. The client is separated or divorced from her husband.

13. The nurse is concerned about abuse within the family unit. Which behavior within the family unit is most consistent with potential abuse?
    1. Participation in numerous activities within the community.
    2. Interaction with a family therapist.
    3. Increased reports of physical illnesses.
    4. Recent weight gain.

14. The nursing assessment reveals the parents of the family in question utilize an authoritative parenting style. Which statement overheard by the nurse when observing interaction between the mother and child confirms this type of parenting style?
    1. "You will do what I tell you to do."
    2. "Let me know when you will be ready to go."
    3. "The decision to participate will be up to you."
    4. "Let's talk about the matter."

15. The mother of a 13-year-old voices concerns about her husband's style of parenting. The mother states her husband allows their teenaged son to make his own rules and seems to avoid confrontation. What parenting style is being described?
    1. Permissive
    2. Persuasive
    3. Dictatorship
    4. Authoritarian

16. The nurse is caring for a 65-year-old female client. Which behavior should alert the nurse to potential abuse? Select all that apply.
    1. Asking numerous questions about the plan of care.
    2. Requesting information about the upcoming discharge.
    3. Inappropriate laughter.
    4. Comments about emotional abuse.

CRITICAL THINKING EXERCISE

Read the case study. Answer the questions, keeping in mind the steps of the nursing process: assessing, diagnosing, planning, implementing, and evaluating.

A nurse is assigned to provide care to two teen clients who are hospitalized in the same room on the pediatric care unit. One family is American Black (African American) and the other is Asian Pacific (Pacific Rim). Both families display allegiance to their cultural traditions. Despite requests of both families to be assigned to another room, none are available on the unit. The nurse is finding it difficult to interact with the families. The families are also experiencing minor conflicts.

1. What should the nurse to do improve their interaction with the families?
2. What knowledge about the cultural beliefs and traditions embraced by the American Black (African American) group will be useful for the nurse during interactions with the client and family?
3. What knowledge about the cultural beliefs and traditions embraced by the Asian Pacific (or Pacific Rim) group will be useful for the nurse during interactions with the client and family?
4. What can be done by the nurse to promote a therapeutic environment within the client room and reduce conflict?

Chapter 4

Reproductive Anatomy and Physiology

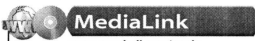

www.prenhall.com/towle

Use the address above to access the free, interactive Companion Website created for this textbook. Get hints, instant feedback to chapter-related NCLEX®-style questions. Link to other interesting sites.

Audio Glossary:

Use the Companion Website, or the CD-ROM disk enclosed with your textbook, to hear the pronunciation of key terms in the chapter.

Care of the childbearing family requires the nurse to have an understanding of the reproductive system of both the male and the female. The nurse's knowledge must include anatomy and physiology, screening tests, and specific health care concerns.

MATCHING

Match the term in the left column with the correct definition in the right column.

1. _____ Gamete
2. _____ Puberty
3. _____ Testes
4. _____ Semen
5. _____ Prostate

6. _____ Prepuce
7. _____ Clitoris
8. _____ Lactogenesis
9. _____ Hymen
10. _____ Oogenesis

A. The production of milk
B. The onset of sexual maturity
C. A thin membrane that partially covers the vaginal orifice
D. A sex cell
E. A doughnut-shaped organ located just below the urinary bladder
F. Development of the female gamete or ovum
G. The essential organ of male reproduction
H. The retractable skin of the penis
I. A mixture of sperm and other fluids produced in the reproductive system
J. Erectile tissue located behind the junction of the labia

FILL IN THE BLANKS

Fill in the blanks with the appropriate word or phrase.

1. Genetic coding is determined by a person's _____.

2. Genetic information is contained in the body's DNA. Four proteins, _____, _____, _____, and _____ compose the DNA.

3. When performing the self-testicular examination, the _____ (spermatic cord), which extends upward toward the base of the penis, is palpated.

4. The number of chromosomes in humans is _____.

5. After the follicle is released from the ovary, the site of expulsion is transformed into the _____, which functions to produce hormones until it gradually degenerates.

6. The _____ of the vagina are mucous membranes that lie in folds. These folds allow the vagina to stretch during a vaginal delivery.

7. A set of glands located on each side of the vagina are responsible for providing lubrication during sexual intercourse. These glands are known as the _____.

8. A pregnant woman notices a thin yellow discharge from her breasts. This fluid is known as _____.

9. The menstrual cycle length lasts an average of 28 days. The phases of each cycle can be divided into three phases: _____, _____, and _____.

10. The physiologic phases in the sexual response cycle are _____, _____, _____, and _____.

MULTIPLE CHOICE

Circle the answer that best completes the following statements.

1. After an educational program about testicular self-examination, which of the following statements made by a participant indicates the need for further instruction?
    1. "I need to begin to perform this examination monthly after I become sexually active."
    2. "Testicular cancer is the most common type of cancer in young men."
    3. "A mirror should be used to assist me in performing the examination."
    4. "If I find any masses, I must report them to my health care provider."

2. The parents of a preteen boy are curious about when their son will be of an age to produce children. Which of the following concepts should be included in the teaching session?
    1. Males have the ability to produce sperm the year prior to puberty.
    2. The ability to father children begins at the close of adolescence.
    3. Males are born with the ability to produce sperm.
    4. Sperm production begins at puberty.

3. An adult male client is concerned about his sex hormone levels. The physical assessment reveals clinical manifestations that may be indicative of a lack of testosterone. Which of the following physical characteristics will support these findings?
   1. Height of less than 5′6″
   2. Thick, curling hair
   3. High-pitched speaking voice
   4. Broad shoulder and chest measurements

4. A laboratory analysis of ejaculate of a male client reveals a reduced amount of fluid produced. Which of the following glands is responsible for a portion of the semen produced? Select all that apply.
   1. Cowper's glands
   2. Penis
   3. Prostate gland
   4. Corpora cavernosa

5. The female client is evaluated for infertility. During the assessment, the client asks when she will produce the eggs needed for reproduction. Which of the following should be included in the nurse's response?
   1. Eggs begin to be produced at puberty.
   2. Egg production begins after the first year of life.
   3. Each female is born with eggs.
   4. The beginning of egg production is variable in each female.

6. The mother of a teenaged female voices concerns that her daughter must not be a virgin because she is able to wear tampons. Which of the following statements by the nurse will be most correct?
   1. "You are probably correct."
   2. "The wearing of a tampon is still possible for someone who has not had sexual intercourse."
   3. "You should consider having your daughter examined by a physician to determine this if you are concerned."
   4. "Have you spoken to your daughter about this matter?"

7. When evaluating the knowledge of a female's ability to perform the breast self-examination, which of the following statements by the client indicates the need for further teaching?
   1. "I will need to begin performing the self-breast exam beginning at puberty."
   2. "Dimpling in my breasts is normal just after my period."
   3. "Standing in front of the mirror will assist me in performing the examination."
   4. "Any breast discharge needs to be reported to my health care provider."

8. A preteen female voices curiosity about the cause of ovulation. Which of the following factors causes this process to take place?
   1. An increase in estrogen
   2. A decrease in progesterone
   3. An increase in follicle stimulating hormone
   4. A peak in the production of luteinizing hormone

9. When preparing to obtain a sexual history from a client, which of the following behaviors by the nurse is most therapeutic?
    1. Ask closed questions to reduce embarrassment.
    2. Ask open-ended questions.
    3. Discuss health promotion practices only if the client indicates an interest to reduce the potential for the client to become uncomfortable.
    4. Require the parent of a teen client to remain in the room to promote open dialogue.

10. The most important purpose for the location of the scrotum is:
    1. Maintain temperature lower than that of the body.
    2. Produce sperm near the point of ejaculation.
    3. Protect the testes and sperm from the effects of the prostate.
    4. Provide room for the convoluted seminiferous tubules.

11. When planning information to be presented at a teaching session concerning the menstrual cycle, which of the following should be included in the presentation?
    1. The failure of menstruation to begin by age 13 requires evaluation.
    2. The menstrual cycle begins on the day of ovulation.
    3. The average length of menstruation is 5 days.
    4. Ovulation occurs in the few days prior to menstruation.

12. Which of the following events is responsible for the onset of menstruation?
    1. An increase in follicle stimulating hormone
    2. An increase in the luteinizing hormone
    3. A reduction in progesterone
    4. An increase in progesterone

13. When a pregnancy results, what processes keep menstruation from occurring?
    1. Increasing levels of progesterone
    2. Destruction of the corpus luteum
    3. Secretion of prolactin
    4. Inhibition of oxytocin production

14. Which of the following statements best describes the labia majora?
    1. It consists of two thin, soft folds of skin, adipose and erectile tissue and covers the vestibule.
    2. It is two folds of skin and adipose tissue covered with hair on either side of the vaginal vestibule and contains sweat and sebaceous glands.
    3. It is a small, erectile body located on the female, containing highly sensitive tissue, and serves a primary role in sexual stimulation for women.
    4. It is the collective term used for the structures of the female reproductive system.

15. After delivery, the changes in which hormone levels are responsible for the change from colostrum to the production of breast milk?
    1. Prolactin
    2. Oxytocin
    3. Estrogen
    4. Progesterone

CRITICAL THINKING EXERCISE

Read the case study. Answer the questions, keeping in mind the steps of the nursing process: assessing, diagnosing, planning, implementing, and evaluating.

The nurse is planning a session to review self-breast examination with teen girls.

1. When is the best time of the month to perform the examination?
2. How do hormones influence the findings of the breast examination?
3. When performing the examination, what positions are recommended?
4. When planning this teaching session, what can the nurse do to reduce feelings of embarrassment?

Chapter 5

Reproductive Issues

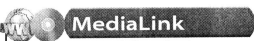

www.prenhall.com/towle

Use the address above to access the free, interactive Companion Website created for this textbook. Get hints, instant feedback to chapter-related NCLEX®-style questions. Link to other interesting sites.

Audio Glossary:

Use the Companion Website, or the CD-ROM disk enclosed with your textbook, to hear the pronunciation of key terms in the chapter.

During their life span, women and men face numerous concerns related to their reproductive health. Ideally, the role of the nurse in relationship to reproductive health needs begins at puberty and extends through the rest of their lives. Included in these reproductive health care needs are health prevention activities, disease screening tests, contraception, and pre- and postnatal care.

MATCHING PART I

Match the term in the left column with the correct definition in the right column.

1. _____ Mammography   A. Painful menses
2. _____ Fibrosis   B. The permanent cessation of menstruation
3. _____ Fibrocyst   C. Noninvasive
4. _____ Fibroadenoma   D. The growth of endometrial tissue outside of the uterus
5. _____ Intraductal papillomas   E. A diagnostic examination of the breast
6. _____ *In situ*   F. The absence of menstruation
7. _____ Mastectomy   G. The growth of tumors in the mammary duct
8. _____ Mammoplasty   H. The replacement of inflamed or damaged tissue with connective scar tissue
9. _____ Dysmenorrhea   I. The removal of a cone-shaped wedge of cervical tissue
10. _____ Menorrhagia   J. Removal of the breast
11. _____ Metrorrhagia   K. Excessive menstrual blood flow
12. _____ Amenorrhea   L. A fluid-filled mass
13. _____ Climacteric   M. Bleeding between menstrual periods
14. _____ Hyperplasia   N. An overgrowth of normal cells

15. _____ Dyspareunia   O.   Reconstruction of the breast

16. _____ Conization   P.   Painful sexual intercourse

17. _____ Endometriosis   Q.   A freely movable rounded mass having well-defined borders

MATCHING PART II

Match the sexually transmitted infection (STI) with the correct corresponding clinical manifestations.

1. _____ Gonorrhea   A.   Fever, malaise, and the appearance of a painless open sore

2. _____ Herpes simplex   B.   Urethritis, purulent urethral drainage, and burning on urination

3. _____ Syphilis   C.   Burning, itching, and the appearance of a painful blister

4. _____ Trichomoniasis   D.   Grayish-pink cauliflower lesions

5. _____ Genital warts   E.   Odorous, frothy, yellow-green discharge

FILL IN THE BLANKS

Fill in the blanks with the appropriate word or phrase.

1. While taking the health history of a 46-year-old client who is having a routine physical examination, the client reports she has not had a menstrual period for the past 18 months. This cessation of menstruation is known as _____.

2. The client in the preceding scenario asks if she has reached this stage prematurely. Based on your knowledge, you report the age in which a woman reaches the climacteric period of her life is _____.

3. When classifying a fibroid tumor of the uterus, the _____ of the tumor will be used.

4. When present, the clinical manifestations of cervical cancer may include _____, _____, and _____. These signs and symptoms signal invasion of the cancer to adjacent structures.

5. A 34-year-old client has been diagnosed with testicular cancer. During preoperative counseling, the client may be advised a(n) _____ incision will be used to remove the diseased testicle.

6. A 16-year-old male reports to the ambulatory health clinic with complaints of pain and swelling in the scrotum, which are worsened with ambulation. A diagnosis of _____ is made.

7. A client wishing to implement herbal remedies to manage his benign prostatic hypertrophy may utilize _____.

MULTIPLE CHOICE

Circle the answer that best completes the following statements.

1. When discussing the onset of menopause with a group of women, which of the following commonly occurring symptoms can be included in the discussion?
    1. Weight loss, hot flashes, feelings of elation
    2. Hot flashes, irritability, and apathy
    3. Apathy, depression, and excessive energy
    4. Moodiness, weight loss, and an increase in appetite

2. A client has been having pain and prolonged periods relating to the presence of several large fibroid tumors in her uterus. After consultation with her gynecologist, the client decides to undergo surgery. The surgery will result in the removal of her uterus. Which of the following terms correctly reflects the name of the procedure that will be performed?
    1. Myomectomy
    2. Exploratory laparotomy
    3. Hysterectomy and bilateral salpingo-oophorectomy
    4. Hysterectomy

3. When reviewing the factors associated with the development of endometrial cancer, which of the following nonmodifiable risk factors may be implicated?
    1. Late menarche and late menopause
    2. Obesity and diabetes
    3. Early menarche and diabetes
    4. Early menopause and the use of oral contraceptives

4. During a community health program, a member of the audience asks you why ovarian cancer is considered the most lethal cancer of the reproductive system. Based upon your knowledge, which of the following is the best response?
    1. "Ovarian cancer is not often detected until it has spread to other parts of the body."
    2. "The number of ovaries a woman has increases this risk."
    3. "The risk factors of this cancer include early menarche and late menopause."
    4. "Few treatment options are available to manage ovarian cancer."

5. At a family support group, a woman states that her sister, who was recently raped, states she is doing fine and has returned to work and school. Her sister asks how that can be possible so soon after such a violent attack. Which of the following should be included in the nurse's best response?
    1. "She must be fine to have returned to her normal schedule."
    2. "Her grief is personal and you must allow her to have some space at this critical time."
    3. "She may be in denial and her rapid return to normalcy are a means for her to establish control."
    4. "Watch her closely for signs of suicidal thoughts."

6. When discussing self-testicular examinations, which of the following findings may be indicative of the disease?
    1. A firm, painful lump
    2. Prostate tenderness with palpation
    3. A hard painless mass
    4. Bilateral testicular tenderness

7. A 66-year-old man reports to the physician's office with complaints of erectile dysfunction. A review of his medical history is performed. Management of which of the following chronic health conditions may be related to this problem? Select all that apply.
    1. Insomnia
    2. Seasonal allergies
    3. Hypertension
    4. Depression
    5. Anxiety

8. When caring for a 17-year-old client who has tested positive for chlamydia, which of the following must be completed before treatment is considered successful?
    1. Education concerning the risk and prevention of reinfection.
    2. Testing for gonorrhea.
    3. Medication therapies that will also treat syphilis.
    4. Follow-up cultures after completion of the prescribed medications.
    5. Identification and testing of sexual contacts.

9. During an appointment for a routine health examination, a client reports she has recently become sexually active. She asks for information concerning available contraceptives. She reports she considers herself spontaneous and dislikes methods that require her to plan ahead for any encounters. Which of the following methods would best meet her needs?
    1. The female condom
    2. IUD
    3. Vaginal diaphragms
    4. Cervical cap

10. The client contacts the clinic with questions regarding the use of her recently fitted vaginal diaphragm. She reports concerns about her diaphragm becoming "lost" or "stuck" after being inserted. Based on your knowledge, which of the following is the best response by the nurse?
    1. "Using the prescribed spermicidal gel will prevent the equipment from becoming stuck in the vaginal cavity."
    2. "The diaphragm can be lodged if left in longer than the recommended 8 hours."
    3. "If the diaphragm becomes stuck in the vaginal cavity, the doctor has a special tool to remove it."
    4. "Your body's structure will not allow the diaphragm to become lost inside you."

11. During her annual pelvic examination, a client reports she has difficulty remembering to take a birth control pill on a daily basis. After further questioning, she states she feels safer using hormonal compounds for contraception. Which of the following methods of contraception would meet the needs of this client? Select all that apply.
    1. The vaginal ring
    2. The contraceptive patch
    3. Female condom
    4. Male condom
    5. Spermicidal gel

12. A woman has undergone a tubal ligation. The LPN/LVN is assisting the RN to plan the discharge teaching. Which of the following must be included in the information given?
    1. The physician will order lab work to determine when the surgery has rendered her infertile.
    2. The procedure is easily reversible should she change her mind.
    3. The woman may immediately engage in sexual intercourse as early as the next day.
    4. The tubal ligation has rendered her infertile upon its completion.

13. A couple reports to the ambulatory clinic. They report being unable to become pregnant after attempting to conceive for the past 3 months. What information should be provided by the nurse?
    1. The couple should be given a listing of tests to evaluate their fertility time.
    2. The couple will benefit from a referral to an infertility specialist.
    3. The couple should be provided information concerning the best days to time sexual relations to promote their ability to conceive a child.
    4. The couple should be given a listing of endocrinologists to make an appointment to have their hormone levels evaluated.

14. A mother brings her teen daughter to the physician's office for her first pelvic examination. The teen has indicated her mother can be involved in her care. During the data collection phase, the mother voices concerns about her daughter's likelihood to engage in sexual activity and become pregnant because many of her friends are having sex and are from an economically disadvantaged background. What information concerning teen pregnancies is correct?
    1. Teens from disadvantaged economic backgrounds are more likely to engage in sexual activity than their more privileged counterparts.
    2. Socioeconomic status has little to no bearing on sexual activity.
    3. Wealthy teens are most likely to engage in early sexual activity.
    4. Education has no impact on pregnancy prevention in teens.

15. During the 6th week of pregnancy, a client experiences complications, and the physician diagnoses an incomplete abortion. Based on your knowledge, which of the following assessment findings can be anticipated?
    1. The cervix will be closed and minimal bleeding evidenced.
    2. The cervix may be slightly open, and the products of conception will be retained.
    3. The fetus is alive, but the pregnancy is in jeopardy with the presence of vaginal bleeding.
    4. The fetus has died and may have been passed, but the placenta has been retained.

CRITICAL THINKING

Read the case study. Answer the questions, keeping in mind the steps of the nursing process: assessing, diagnosing, planning, implementing, and evaluating.

A 31-year-old client has been notified by her primary care physician of irregularities in her annual Pap smear. The client has been diagnosed with cervical dysplasia. Based on your knowledge, respond to the following questions.

1. What topical information should be provided to the client concerning this diagnosis?
2. List risk factors associated with the development of cervical dysplasia.
3. What treatment options are available for the client diagnosed with cervical dysplasia?
4. Review the relationship between cervical dysplasia and cervical cancer.

Chapter 6

Health Promotion During Pregnancy

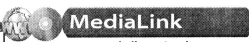

MediaLink

www.prenhall.com/towle

Use the address above to access the free, interactive Companion Website created for this textbook. Get hints, instant feedback to chapter-related NCLEX®-style questions. Link to other interesting sites.

Audio Glossary:

Use the Companion Website, or the CD-ROM disk enclosed with your textbook, to hear the pronunciation of key terms in the chapter.

The health and wellness of the baby at the time of birth are in large part determined by the care received by the mother during her pregnancy. A woman's preparations for pregnancy should ideally begin prior to conception. After the woman becomes pregnant, early prenatal care and other health promotion activities can increase the likelihood of a positive birth outcome.

MATCHING

Match the term in the left column with the correct definition in the right column.

1. _____ Anomalies
2. _____ Teratogens
3. _____ Salpingitis
4. _____ Fertilization
5. _____ Zygote
6. _____ Morula
7. _____ Blastocyst
8. _____ Trophoblast
9. _____ Lanugo
10. _____ Vernix caseosa
11. _____ Cotyledons
12. _____ Wharton's jelly
13. _____ Cephalocaudal

A. Infection of the fallopian tubes

B. A substance responsible for reducing surface tension in the alveoli

C. White gelatinous material that surrounds the umbilical cord

D. Abnormal organ or structure development

E. A two-layer ball of cells

F. Fine hair covering the fetus

G. Drugs or other agents that may cause abnormal fetal development

H. White, cheesy covering of the fetal skin

I. Irregular sections of the maternal side of the placenta

J. The union of the sperm and the ovum

K. The term used to refer to the fertilized egg

L. A multicelled mulberry-shaped mass

M. Occurring from head to toe

14. _____ Surfactant   N.   The ability of the fetus to survive outside the uterus

15. _____ Viability   O.   The outer layer of the blastocyst

FILL IN THE BLANKS

Fill in the blanks with the appropriate word or phrase.

1. After the sperm are released in the woman's body, they travel to meet the ovum. In most cases these sex cells unite in the _____.

2. After conception, the fertilized egg travels to the uterus, where _____ results.

3. A client prepares to take a home pregnancy test. The test is positive. The chemical that is found in the urine to signal pregnancy is known as _____.

4. The fluid that surrounds the fetus is predominately water. Other substances in this fluid include _____, _____, _____, _____, and _____.

5. The period of time in which the egg is fertilized by the sperm and it travels to the uterus and attaches to the endometrium is known as _____.

6. After waste products are removed from the blood, the oxygenated blood and nutrients are returned to the fetus via the _____.

7. The fetal production of bile when combined with amniotic fluid and epithelial cells forms _____.

8. The stages of the pregnancy are recorded in three-month blocks of time known as _____.

9. A client has noted her facial coloring has changed during her pregnancy. The assessment reveals her forehead, cheeks and the area around her eyes are darker. This change in pigmentation is known as _____.

MULTIPLE CHOICE

Circle the answer that best completes the following statements.

1. A couple who is actively trying to conceive a child has an appointment at the ambulatory clinic. During their appointment, the woman states that she has discontinued smoking cigarettes and drinking alcohol and has begun taking numerous herbal preparations in planning for her pregnancy. What is the best response by the nurse at this time?
   1. "You should be commended for taking such an active role in your health care."
   2. "The herbal supplements will be more effective if taken at bedtime."
   3. "Herbal remedies are beneficial to women during the pregnancy."
   4. "Any medications and herbal supplements may interfere with the pregnancy and should be discussed with your physician."

2. A client calls the clinic to ask about the use of home pregnancy tests. She asks when her physical changes will signal a positive test. Based on your knowledge, what information should be included in the teaching plan? Select all that apply.
   1. The body will begin to produce HCG within 8 to 10 days after fertilization.
   2. The urine test will become positive sooner than the blood test.
   3. Urine testing is unreliable for the first 11 to 12 weeks.
   4. Urine testing may be done at home a few days prior to the expected menstrual period.
   5. The HCG is produced by the chorionic villi.

3. During a routine prenatal care appointment, a client voices concerns about the placenta's blood flow. She asks if there can be problems with compatibility because her blood is flowing into the baby via the placenta. What information will guide the nurse's response?
   1. The blood type of the mother and baby are the same and thus compatible.
   2. The blood cells of the mother and fetus are not directly exchanged.
   3. There are significant risks due to the exchange process between the mother and the fetus.
   4. The fetus has specialized immunoglobulin cells to provide protection from the maternal blood cells.

4. While attending a prenatal education class, a parent asks how the woman's body is able to accommodate the increase in fetal weight. What is the best explanation for the phenomena?
   1. Hormones are produced to assist the mother's joints to relax and accommodate the body's growing changes.
   2. The increase in cardiac output enables the body to handle the size increases associated with pregnancy.
   3. Estrogen promotes elasticity in the body vessels.
   4. Human chorionic gonadotropin is used by the body to relax the joints.

5. A mother preparing for admission to the hospital for a scheduled cesarean section asks the nurse what prevents significant blood loss from the cord after delivery. Which of the following statements best answers her query?
   1. The physician will cauterize the vessels to prevent excessive blood loss after delivery.
   2. During the delivery, the cord ceases to function and prevents significant blood loss.
   3. Closure of the ductus arteriosis prevents excessive bleeding.
   4. Environmental changes have a unique effect on the umbilical cord rendering it incapable of significant blood loss.

6. While at their first prenatal care visit, the client's husband asks when the baby's sex will be determined. The client is presently at 7 weeks gestation. What information should be provided to the couple regarding this matter? Select all that apply.
   1. Sex is determined at the time of conception.
   2. The baby's sex can be distinguished as early as the 12th week of gestation.
   3. Sperm will not be produced until puberty.
   4. A "Y" chromosome fertilizing the egg will result in the development of a female child.
   5. If an "X" chromosome fertilized the egg, a male child will develop.
   6. A transvaginal ultrasound performed today can distinguish the fetus' gender.

7. After the delivery of a preterm infant, the African American parents are distressed because their baby's skin is very pale and pink. What will best explain this occurrence?
   1. The thin, pink skin is a result the lack of fat present in a premature infant.
   2. The child must have a light complexion.
   3. There is an inadequate amount of blood flow resulting in the reduction of skin color.
   4. Pallor is normal in newborns due to thermoregulation difficulties.

8. A woman is seen at the physician's office. She states she has experienced signs and symptoms consistent with being pregnant. She reports feeling nauseated, and her menstrual period is 4 days late. Despite these manifestations the pregnancy test is negative. What can explain the inconsistency between these findings?
   1. The symptoms reported are only probable and may not be considered definitive.
   2. The symptoms being reported are not considered diagnostic and may be attributed to other conditions.
   3. It is too early in the pregnancy for a urine HCG test to be positive.
   4. The symptoms being experienced are most likely due to stress or illness.

9. When assessing the fetal heart tones using the Doppler, the rate is found to be 120 beats per minute. What action is indicated next?
   1. Document the findings.
   2. Do nothing.
   3. Notify the physician.
   4. Schedule an ultrasound.

10. During her 31st week of pregnancy, a client reports she felt dizzy after lying down for a nap. What additional information should be collected by the nurse to assist in determining the underlying cause for her symptoms?
    1. The position she used while resting.
    2. The time of day the symptoms were experienced.
    3. The length of time she laid down for the nap.
    4. What she did after experiencing these symptoms.

11. The complete blood cell count for a client in her 29th week of pregnancy reflects a hemoglobin of 12.1. What is the most likely cause for this finding?
    1. The client is not taking the prescribed iron supplements.
    2. The client's nutritional intake is not adequate.
    3. Additional tests will be needed to determine the underlying cause of these findings.
    4. The increase in red blood cells has not kept pace with the increase in circulating blood volume.

12. At her first prenatal appointment a 41-year-old woman voices concerns about her upcoming amniocentesis. She is currently 9 weeks gestation and does not understand why she cannot have the test moved up to the following week. Explain the rationale for not completing this test during the first trimester.
    1. The fetus will not be large enough to examine using the amniocentesis until that time.
    2. The placenta will not provide adequate information until the second trimester.
    3. There is not adequate amniotic fluid to perform the test until after the 15th week of gestation.
    4. The risk of fetal loss is too great until the second trimester.

13. A teenaged client has developed numerous "stretch marks." She is concerned about their appearance. She asks questions about their prognosis. What will be included in the information provided?
    1. These marks will disappear in the weeks following delivery of the baby.
    2. Stretch marks will disappear if cocoa butter is used on a daily basis during the entire pregnancy.
    3. The more weight gained, the more difficult it will be to get rid of these marks.
    4. These marks will fade but will not go away.

14. A 22-year-old woman reported to the clinic and had a positive pregnancy test performed. During the data collection she advised the nurse her last normal menstrual period was May 15th. This menstrual cycle lasted until May 19th. Based on your knowledge, what will the estimated date of delivery be?
    1. February 8th
    2. February 22nd
    3. February 26th
    4. February 12th

15. A woman in her 29th week of pregnancy is hospitalized. She has concerns relating to body image and has begun dieting. Her weight has decreased 9 pounds over the past 3 weeks. After completing the shift assessment, the LPN/LVN is assisting the RN to develop a nursing care plan. Which of the following potential nursing diagnoses is of the highest priority at the time of admission?
    1. Deficient Knowledge Related to the Nutritional Needs of the Fetus
    2. Body Image Disturbance
    3. Nutrition: Altered, Less Than Body Requirements
    4. Constipation

CRITICAL THINKING EXERCISE

Read the case study. Answer the questions, keeping in mind the steps of the nursing process: assessing, diagnosing, planning, implementing, and evaluating.

A client has reported to the clinic for a routinely scheduled prenatal care appointment. During the examination, she reports feeling constipated.

1. What factors associated with pregnancy can explain this condition?
2. What interventions can be implemented to reduce this occurrence?
3. Discuss the use of medications to manage the client's constipation.
4. Discuss the use of enemas to manage the client's constipation.

Chapter 7

Health Promotion During Labor and Delivery

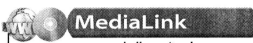

www.prenhall.com/towle

Use the address above to access the free, interactive Companion Website created for this textbook. Get hints, instant feedback to chapter-related NCLEX®-style questions. Link to other interesting sites.

Audio Glossary:

Use the Companion Website, or the CD-ROM disk enclosed with your textbook, to hear the pronunciation of key terms in the chapter.

Labor and delivery is greatly anticipated by the family expecting the birth of a child. Preparation of the client is best when it begins before onset of labor. The client requires education concerning what will be taking place to prepare her body for the upcoming labor. The signs and symptoms of labor and when to seek care should be included in the planned teaching. During labor the role of the nurse involves meeting both the physical and emotional needs of the client.

MATCHING

Match the term in the left column with the correct definition in the right column.

1. _____ Lightening
   A. Relationship of the fetal presenting part to the maternal ischial spines

2. _____ Effacement
   B. Performed to assess for the presence of amniotic fluid

3. _____ Dilatation
   C. Descent of the fetus into the maternal pelvis

4. _____ Episiotomy
   D. An incision to increase the diameter of vaginal opening

5. _____ Nitrazine test
   E. Softening and thinning of the cervix

6. _____ Amniotomy
   F. Widening in diameter of the cervix

7. _____ Station
   G. Artificial rupture of membranes

8. _____ Fetal attitude
   H. Shaping of the fetal head to the bones of the maternal pelvis

9. _____ Fetal lie
   I. The relationship of the body parts to each other

10. _____ Molding
   J. The relationship of the long axis of the fetus to the long axis of the mother

FILL IN THE BLANKS

Fill in the blanks with the appropriate word or phrase.

1. A client has reported to the hospital. She reports she has been experiencing "abdominal cramps." The nurse in the labor and delivery department performs an assessment and determines the client is having false labor. What term is used to describe these pains? _____

2. During her 39th week of pregnancy, a client notes a blood-tinged mucous discharge from her vagina. The client consults the nurse. The nurse advises the client _____ is the release of the mucous plug from the cervix.

3. A client in her 32nd week of pregnancy reports to the hospital. The RN performs an assessment. The LPN/LVN understands the client's "water has broken." This condition is known as _____.

4. During a routinely scheduled prenatal care appointment, the health care provider has performed an assessment of the client's pelvis. It has been determined the fetal head is too large to be safely accommodated by the mother's pelvis. This condition is known as _____.

5. A vaginal assessment is performed on a client in her 36th week of pregnancy. The assessment reveals the fetus is cephalic. The term used to refer to the positioning of the fetus is known as the _____.

6. During the active phase of labor, the client is sitting in Fowler's position and stroking her abdomen. This technique is known as _____.

7. In the _____ phase of labor, the onset of contractions will begin and the cervix will dilate to 4 cm.

8. After delivery, the occurrence of a gush of blood from the vagina and lengthening of the umbilical cord from the vagina are signs of _____.

9. Expulsion of the placenta with the maternal side out is known as _____.

10. After an examination by the physician, it is determined the fetus is presenting with the buttocks presenting first. This type of presentation is known as _____.

MULTIPLE CHOICE

Circle the answer that best completes the following statements.

1. During a routinely scheduled prenatal care visit, a client reports that she has been noticing a need to void more frequently during the past week. She wonders if she is developing a urinary tract infection. Further history taking and assessment by the nurse reveals the client, who is at 37 weeks gestation, is also experiencing increased fatigue, lower leg edema, and leg cramps. Which of the following responses by the nurse is most appropriate?
   1. "You have a bladder infection."
   2. "Drinking more fluids will assist with these discomforts."

3. "You are experiencing discomforts related to your baby's descent into the pelvis."

4. "You will probably go into labor in the next 2 weeks."

2. The client is in her 38th week of pregnancy. She experiences the rupture of her membranes. Concerned, she contacts the medical center. Which of the following instructions should be given to the client by the nurse?

1. The client should be advised to report to the medical center for further evaluation.

2. The client should be advised to ambulate for a period of time at home and come in only if contractions begin.

3. The client should be advised to put on a sanitary pad and monitor the discharge at home for 60 minutes.

4. The client should be instructed to remain at home until a regular contraction pattern begins.

3. The client with ruptured membranes is admitted to the labor and delivery unit. The assessment reveals the client is in her 39th week of gestation. Which of the following statements by the client reveals the need for further teaching?

1. "I will be discharged if my labor does not begin within 24 hours."

2. "I am excited about becoming a mother."

3. "My baby is finally going to be born."

4. "I will be giving birth to my child during this hospital admission."

4. An assessment on the client in labor is completed. Which of the fetal positions will most likely require a cesarean section delivery?

1. Mentum presentation

2. Vertex presentation

3. Face presentation

4. Breech presentation

5. The nurse performs a vaginal examination on the client suspected to be in labor. The examination reveals the client is dilated 5 cm and is 75% effaced. Which of the following can be determined by the vaginal examination? Select all that apply.

1. Sex of the fetus

2. Fetal presenting part

3. Strength of contraction pattern

4. Gestational age of the fetus

6. A vaginal examination is performed on the client who is at term. Which of the findings indicates the client is experiencing false labor?

1. Contractions that increase in intensity with ambulation.

2. Contractions felt in the abdomen above the umbilicus.

3. Contractions felt in the lower back and radiating to the lower portion of the abdomen.

4. Movement of the cervix into an increasingly anterior position.

7. During the prenatal education class, there is a presentation concerning the use of doulas. Which of the following statements by the pregnant client reflect the need for further teaching? Select all that apply.
   1. "When my husband and I hire a doula for our birthing experience, she will communicate my needs and desires to the physician."
   2. "Doula use is associated with positive outcomes such as shorter labors and reduced cesarean sections."
   3. "The doula will manage my care when my nurse is on break."
   4. "Women who have doulas do not require pain medication during labor."

8. Upon admission to the labor and delivery unit, a health assessment and physical examination are completed. Which of the following questions asked of the client assist the nurse to determine the progression/length of the client's labor? Select all that apply.
   1. What was the length of the client's mother's labor?
   2. What is the number of years since the client's last labor?
   3. When did the contractions begin?
   4. Have the membranes ruptured?

9. When providing culturally sensitive care to the client of South Korean descent, knowledge of which of the following potential health beliefs may be beneficial?
   1. A preference for female caregivers.
   2. Stoic during labor.
   3. The desire to have both the father of the baby and their own father present for the labor and delivery.
   4. The desire to have hot food and warm water available during labor.

10. A client in the later stages of labor requests a diet cola. Which of the responses by the nurses is most appropriate?
   1. "A non-diet cola would be best at this time as it will provide you with glucose for energy."
   2. "I will get that for you to drink between contractions."
   3. "At this stage of your labor, ice chips would be best due to the risk of vomiting."
   4. "You can have something after your baby is born."

11. One minute after birth, the neonate's Apgar score is 8. Which of the following interventions by the nurse is indicated at this time?
   1. Narcan should be administered to the neonate.
   2. The infant's back should be rubbed to stimulate a more effective breathing pattern.
   3. Document the findings.
   4. Flick the soles of the infant's feet to increase the respiratory efforts.

12. The client is in labor. The client tells the nurse the physician has indicated plans to rupture her membranes. Which of the following statements by the nurse indicates an understanding of the planned procedure?
   1. "I will deliver shortly after the physician ruptures my membranes."
   2. "I am nervous about having a dry birth."
   3. "The physician will give me some medication to cause my water to break."
   4. "Breaking my water may speed up my labor."

13. While caring for a client who is in the transition phase of labor and dilated to 9 cm, the client states, "I am ready to push." Which of the responses by the nurse is most appropriate?
    1. "Push between contractions."
    2. "To increase the force delivered, push while holding your breath."
    3. "Let's focus on your breathing techniques to avoid pushing right now."
    4. "Roll onto your side to reduce the urge to push."

14. After the birth of the baby, the nurse is performing an assessment on the neonate. Which of the following findings indicates the need for further actions by the nurse?
    1. Vernix is present.
    2. The umbilical cord has one artery and one vein.
    3. The umbilical cord has two arteries and one vein.
    4. Palmar creases are present.

15. While caring for the client in the first hour after delivery, which of the findings is anticipated?
    1. Blood loss of approximately 750 mL
    2. An increase in blood pressure
    3. Gradual decrease in heart rate
    4. Tachycardia

CRITICAL THINKING EXERCISE

Read the case study. Answer the questions, keeping in mind the steps of the nursing process: assessing, diagnosing, planning, implementing, and evaluating.

A client is admitted to the labor and delivery unit. The nursing assessment reveals the client is in early labor. The cervical assessment reveals dilatation at 3 cm and 70% effaced. The client voices feelings of anxiety about the pain she may experience. She reports she discussed this with her physician but is having difficulty remembering all the details. She asks you for additional information.

1. The client is interested in information about the epidural. What are the advantages of having an epidural? What are disadvantages?

2. If the client has an epidural, what are potential side effects the nurse must be aware of?

3. The client asks the nurse about being "knocked out" if the pain becomes too much for her to handle. How should the nurse respond?

4. After listening to the information provided by the nurse, the client decides to have systemic medications. How are these medications given? When in the labor process can these medications be given?

Chapter 8

Maternal High-Risk Nursing Care

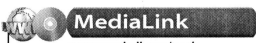

MediaLink

www.prenhall.com/towle

Use the address above to access the free, interactive Companion Website created for this textbook. Get hints, instant feedback to chapter-related NCLEX®-style questions. Link to other interesting sites.

Audio Glossary:

Use the Companion Website, or the CD-ROM disk enclosed with your textbook, to hear the pronunciation of key terms in the chapter.

Pregnancy is generally a time of wellness; however, a pregnancy may be classified as high risk. It is the responsibility of the nurse providing care to the pregnant woman to have knowledge of potential complications and treatment and management of these complications that may result during pregnancy, in labor, and in the postpartum phase.

MATCHING

Match the term in the left column with the correct definition in the right column.

1. _____ Ultrasound
2. _____ Amniocentesis
3. _____ Nonstress test
4. _____ Ectopic pregnancy
5. _____ Indirect Coombs' test
6. _____ Abruptio placenta
7. _____ Threatened abortion
8. _____ Dystocia
9. _____ Inevitable abortion
10. _____ Hyperemesis gravidarum

A. Bleeding and cramping with cervical dilation
B. Used to assess heart rate in relation to fetal movement
C. Bleeding and cramping with cervical closure
D. A long, difficult, or abnormal labor pattern
E. Implantation of the fertilized egg outside the uterus
F. Premature separation of the placenta from the uterine wall
G. The use of sound waves used to visualize maternal and fetal structures
H. A condition characterized by excessive nauseas and vomiting during pregnancy
I. A blood test used to assess maternal sensitization to fetal blood cells
J. The withdrawal of amniotic fluid through a needle inserted into the abdomen and the uterus

FILL IN THE BLANKS

Fill in the blanks with the appropriate word or phrase.

1. A mother's Rh factor is negative and her fetus's blood is Rh positive. If the antibodies from the fetus cross into the maternal circulation, a condition known as _____ may result.

2. When assisting a mother to the recommended therapeutic position to perform a nonstress test, positioning the mother in _____ is done.

3. An assessment of fetal condition may be achieved by performing a biophysical profile. The variables reviewed in a biophysical profile include _____, _____, _____, _____, and _____.

4. At 6 weeks gestation, a client is advised her baby has died. The physician explains to the client that a surgical procedure will be indicated to remove the products of conception from the uterus. The procedure being discussed is known as _____.

5. After experiencing three consecutive miscarriages in 2 years, a client has been scheduled to undergo a surgical procedure designed to prevent premature dilation of the cervix. The procedure the client will face is known as a _____.

6. The client presents with painless vaginal bleeding during her third trimester of pregnancy. The complication of pregnancy associated with the preceding clinical manifestations is known as _____.

7. While performing an assessment on a client who is 30 weeks pregnant, you note the following clinical manifestations: edema in the hands and face, hyper reflexes, and a blood pressure of 144/92. These findings are indicative of _____.

8. The postpartum assessment includes an evaluation of vaginal bleeding. The three primary reasons for postpartum hemorrhage include: _____, _____, and _____.

MULTIPLE CHOICE

Circle the answer that best completes the following statements.

1. A client has a high-risk condition that makes preterm delivery a probable occurrence. An amniocentesis has been performed. When reviewing the results, which of the results indicate the fetus has lung maturity to enable the fetus to avoid significant respiratory compromise?
   1. Lecithin/sphingomyelin ratio at 1:2
   2. Lecithin/sphingomyelin ratio at 2:1
   3. Absence of phosphatidylglycerol
   4. Equal amounts of lecithin, sphingomyelin, and phosphatidylglycerol

2. A client is scheduled to have a nonstress test performed. The LPN/LVN will have which of the following roles related to this task? Select all that apply.
   1. The LPN/LVN will be responsible for assisting the client into the correct position.
   2. The LPN/LVN will secure the equipment to the mother to perform the test.
   3. The LPN/LVN will interpret the results of the test after completion.
   4. The LPN/LVN will remove the recording equipment after the test is completed.

3. After the biophysical profile is performed, the client receives a score of 9. Which of the following can be discerned from these results?
   1. The baby will most likely be born via cesarean section.
   2. The baby does not exhibit any outward signs of distress.
   3. Follow up with an oxytocin challenge test is indicated.
   4. The baby is in fetal distress.

4. A client at 25 weeks gestation undergoes a 1-hour glucose screening test. The results of the test indicate a test value of 132 mg/dL. Which of the following is the best interpretation of these results?
   1. The client has diabetes mellitus type 1.
   2. The client has demonstrated a normal blood glucose value for this period of gestation.
   3. This result indicates the need of further evaluation of the client's status.
   4. The client has diabetes mellitus type 2.

5. A client has a positive pregnancy test after her period is 2 days late. The following day, the client begins to experience a small amount of vaginal bleeding. Which of the following statements is correct concerning this client's condition? Select all that apply.
   1. The client is experiencing placenta previa.
   2. The client is experiencing an inevitable abortion.
   3. The pregnancy may continue if the blastocyst remains attached to the endometrial lining of the uterus.
   4. The levels of HCG may not be high enough to prevent the bleeding's occurrence.

6. While providing postoperative care to a client who has just experienced her fourth pregnancy loss, the client states she is a failure as a woman and is unable to carry a child to term. Which of the following is the most therapeutic response by the nurse?
   1. "I know how you feel."
   2. "You are not alone, there is another client, Mary, in room 102, who has just lost her baby as well."
   3. "Tell me more about how you are feeling."
   4. "Is your family there for you to discuss these feelings?"

7. A client had a positive serum pregnancy test 4 days after the first missed pregnancy. One week later, the client has begun to experience severe abdominal pain and a moderate amount of vaginal bleeding. The physician diagnosed the presence of an ectopic pregnancy in her left fallopian tube. The client is tearful

and later asks why her baby cannot be saved. Which of the following is the best response to the client?

1. "I understand you are sad but you will have more children."
2. "The baby's growth will be stopped by the confines of your fallopian tube and will cause damage if not removed."
3. "There are experimental treatments that will allow you to continue this pregnancy."
4. "You may die if the physician does not treat you."

8. A client presents to the labor and delivery department with complaints of painless vaginal bleeding. Which of the following activities are contraindicated?
   1. A vaginal examination
   2. Ultrasound
   3. Nonstress test
   4. Biophysical profile

9. A client at 31 weeks gestation has been diagnosed with total placenta previa. After a brief hospitalization, she is preparing to be discharged to home. Which of the following statements by the client indicates the need for further education?
   1. "I will need to contact my employer about my inability to return to my waitress job."
   2. "I can't wait to experience my baby's birth vaginally."
   3. "I will need to remain on bedrest indefinitely."
   4. "If my bleeding worsens, I will need to seek medical care."

10. A client at 34 weeks gestation has been admitted to the hospital after being involved in a motor vehicle crash. After admission the client was assessed and an ultrasound performed. The client was diagnosed with a centrally located placenta previa. Which of the following clinical manifestations would be anticipated?
    1. Perfuse vaginal bleeding and severe abdominal pain
    2. Minimal vaginal bleeding and abdominal pain
    3. Moderate vaginal bleeding and no abdominal pain
    4. Absence of vaginal bleeding and significant abdominal pain

11. Which of the following clients has the greatest risk for developing puerperal infection?
    1. A primigravida who has experienced a vaginal delivery.
    2. A client who has delivered her child via cesarean section and her membranes were ruptured for 18 hours.
    3. The multigravida who has just vaginally delivered twins.
    4. The client who has a scheduled cesarean section for a breech presentation.

12. The LPN/LVN is assigned to a client on the antepartum unit with a diagnosis of placenta previa. Which of the following potential nursing diagnoses is appropriate and of the highest priority for the client?
    1. Deficient Knowledge, Related to High-Risk Pregnancy
    2. Anxiety
    3. Tissue Perfusion, Ineffective
    4. Activity Intolerance

13. A client arrives at the labor and delivery unit stating, "The baby is coming right now." As you assist the client to the bed, it becomes apparent delivery is imminent. List in order the steps that must be taken to ensure a safe progression for the client and her baby.
    1. Check the baby's neck for the umbilical cord.
    2. Suction the baby's mouth.
    3. Tear the membranes.
    4. Apply gentle pressure to head.

14. The client has been hospitalized to treat preterm labor. The client is presently 29 weeks gestation. Which of the following statements by the client indicates the need for further teaching?
    1. "I must have a cesarean to deliver my child because of his prematurity."
    2. "The medications I take to stop my preterm labor contractions may cause my heart to beat rapidly."
    3. "There are medications that can be used to help speed the maturation of my baby's lungs."
    4. "My preterm labor may be associated with my history of repeated vaginal infections."

15. While working on the postpartum unit, you are assigned to provide care to four clients. Which of the following clients is a candidate to receive RhoGAM?
    1. A mother who is Rh negative who has given birth to a baby who is Rh negative.
    2. A mother who is Rh positive who has given birth to a baby who is Rh positive.
    3. A mother who is Rh positive who has given birth to a baby who is Rh negative.
    4. A mother who is Rh negative who has given birth to a baby who is Rh positive.

CRITICAL THINKING EXERCISE

Read the case study. Answer the questions, keeping in mind the steps of the nursing process: assessing, diagnosing, planning, implementing, and evaluating.

A client reports to the labor room. She is tearful and advises the nurse she has not felt her baby move for more than 24 hours. A health history assessment reveals the client is 34 weeks pregnant and has had an uneventful pregnancy thus far.

1. What testing can be anticipated to determine the status of the fetus?
2. If the fetus has expired in utero, what term is used to describe this event?
3. Discuss the role of the significant other or support person.
4. If deceased, when and how will the delivery take place?
5. Discuss care that should be provided to the client after delivery of the baby.

Chapter 9

Health Promotion of the Newborn

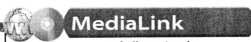

www.prenhall.com/towle

Use the address above to access the free, interactive Companion Website created for this textbook. Get hints, instant feedback to chapter-related NCLEX®-style questions. Link to other interesting sites.

Audio Glossary:

Use the Companion Website, or the CD-ROM disk enclosed with your textbook, to hear the pronunciation of key terms in the chapter.

During the transition from gestation to birth, the infant experiences multiple changes. The role of the nurse in caring for newborns focuses on assessment of appropriate adaptation to extrauterine life. The nurse has many assessment areas to evaluate during the newborn period. Teaching for the parents/caregivers occurs frequently during this short time frame. Having an understanding of basic variations of the newborn is necessary for determining priority nursing actions.

MATCHING

Match the term in the left column with the correct definition in the right column.

1. _____ Meconium
2. _____ Acrocyanosis
3. _____ Nonshivering thermogenesis
4. _____ Petechiae
5. _____ Lanugo
6. _____ Milia
7. _____ Cephalhematoma
8. _____ Apgar score
9. _____ Ecchymosis
10. _____ Caput succedaneum

A. Fine downy hair covering a newborn
B. Enlarged sebaceous glands on the face
C. Bruising after delivery
D. Method of evaluating a newborn's adaptation in the first few minutes of life
E. Edema of the scalp
F. Bluish discoloration of hands and feet
G. The blackish green first stool of a newborn
H. Heat generated by burning stored brown fat
I. Accumulation of blood under the skull bone
J. Pinpoint hemorrhages

FILL IN THE BLANKS

Fill in the blanks with the appropriate word or phrase.

1. A new mother needs to add _____ to _____ extra calories to her diet when breastfeeding.

2. _____ is the first fluid produced by the breast and is a thin _____ fluid that is easily digested by the newborn.

3. A newborn will usually _____ weight during the first few days of life.

4. The newborn should pass _____ stool within the first _____ hours of life.

5. A newborn should be placed _____ _____ _____ in the crib to sleep.

6. A major priority to observe for following a circumcision is _____.

7. One site that may be used to administer intravenous fluids to a newborn is in a(n) _____ _____.

8. Newborns born to mothers who have a history of gonorrhea and herpes need to be delivered by _____ _____.

9. An infant born before _____ weeks gestation is at risk for hemorrhage in the brain known as _____ _____.

10. Cyanosis that is observed around the newborn's mouth would be documented as _____ _____.

MULTIPLE CHOICE

Circle the answer that best completes the following statements.

1. Which of the following methods are appropriate when stimulating newborn breathing just after birth? Select all that apply.
   1. Use of an Ambu bag-valve mask
   2. Rubbing the skin
   3. Application of oxygen
   4. Slapping the buttocks
   5. Tapping the soles of the feet

2. Which of the following methods are appropriate when preventing heat loss in a newborn immediately after birth? Select all that apply.
   1. Applying a hat
   2. Place newborn next to mother
   3. Wrap in warm blankets
   4. Give a quick initial bath
   5. Dry with warm blankets

3. A newborn with which Apgar score at 5 minutes of age would need closer assessment and observation.
   1. 10
   2. 9
   3. 8
   4. 7

4. Jaundice of the skin is a result of:
   1. Intolerance to breast milk.
   2. Immature intestinal system.
   3. Bilirubin accumulation in the blood.
   4. Low number of circulating red blood cells.

5. A mother notices several "rash" areas over her newborn's chest and abdomen at 24 hours of age. A common cause of this is:
   1. Caput succedaneum.
   2. Cephalhematoma.
   3. Milia.
   4. Erythema toxicum neonatorum.

6. When removing a newborn's hat for the first time, the father is upset to find the head is cone-shaped. This results from positioning in the mother's pelvis known as:
   1. Molding.
   2. Vernix caseosa.
   3. Edema.
   4. Perfusion.

7. A major difference between caput succedaneum and cephalhematoma is that:
   1. Caput succedaneum will not cross suture lines.
   2. Cephalhematoma occurs from molding.
   3. Caput succedaneum may cross suture lines.
   4. Caput succedaneum is from bleeding in the head.

8. An early sign of respiratory distress in a newborn would be:
   1. Retracting.
   2. Nasal flaring.
   3. Wheezing.
   4. Expiratory grunting.

9. When retracting is noted suprasternally, the nurse knows that this is a sign that the:
   1. Respiratory status is stabilizing.
   2. Respiratory status is worsening.
   3. Newborn is stabile enough to bathe.
   4. Newborn is stabile enough to eat.

10. A nurse is concerned when a chart is accidentally dropped next to a newborn's crib and the awake infant does not move. Which response would the nurse have anticipated?
    1. Crying
    2. Babinski response
    3. Stepping movement
    4. Abduction of arms

11. Antibiotic ointment is placed in a newborn's eyes soon after delivery to:
    1. Help the newborn sleep.
    2. Prevent ophthalmia neonatorum.
    3. Prevent hemorrhage disorders.
    4. Help eyes focus on parents.

12. Vitamin K (aqua Mephyton) is given by which route within 1 hour after delivery?
    1. Orally
    2. Intramuscularly
    3. Subcutaneously
    4. Topically

13. During a teaching session for bathing, the nurse will point out that the newborn may have a tub bath:
    1. Once they get home.
    2. When they gain 2 pounds.
    3. After the cord falls off.
    4. After the first physician's visit.

14. Small gestational age (SGA) or large gestational age (LGA) newborns are closely monitored for:
    1. Jaundice.
    2. Phenylketonuria (PKU).
    3. Hypoglycemia.
    4. Acrocyanosis.

15. A primipara mother is upset that she is having difficulty breastfeeding her newborn in the first day of life. The nurse's best response would be:
    1. Report the problem to the doctor.
    2. Offer to stay with her during the next feeding.
    3. Suggest that she switch to bottle feeding.
    4. Give her a pamphlet discussing breastfeeding.

CRITICAL THINKING EXERCISE

Read the case study. Answer the questions, keeping in mind the steps of the nursing process: assessing, diagnosing, planning, implementing, and evaluating.

A newborn is delivered at 35 weeks gestation by emergency cesarean section. This is the parent's first baby. No sonogram had been done prenatally. A unilateral cleft lip and palate are noted upon delivery. At 18 hours of age, the newborn's skin is noted to be slightly jaundiced. You are the LPN/LVN working with the RN to provide care for this newborn and parents. You begin your planning by answering the following questions.

1. Discuss the priority assessment needs immediately after birth for this newborn.

2. Discuss the involvement of the parents with this newborn.

3. Review the mother's history to determine any prenatal influences on this newborn's situation and what action would be taken first.

4. Identify long-term potential and actual problems that will involve teaching by the nurse.

Chapter 10

Health Promotion in the Postpartum Period

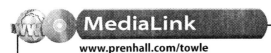
www.prenhall.com/towle

Use the address above to access the free, interactive Companion Website created for this textbook. Get hints, instant feedback to chapter-related NCLEX®-style questions. Link to other interesting sites.

Audio Glossary:

Use the Companion Website, or the CD-ROM disk enclosed with your textbook, to hear the pronunciation of key terms in the chapter.

After the birth of the baby, the family dynamics are altered. The mother of the baby will experience the physiological and psychological changes associated with the postpartum period. Nursing care and teaching are essential to assist the mother during this period of transition.

MATCHING

Match the term in the left column with the correct definition in the right column.

1. _____ Puerperium

2. _____ Involution

3. _____ Prolactin

4. _____ Hematoma

5. _____ Engorgement

6. _____ RhoGAM

7. _____ Diastasis recti abdominis

8. _____ Oxytocin

9. _____ Mastitis

10. _____ Bonding

A. An accumulation of blood under the skin

B. Hormone produced by the anterior pituitary gland responsible for milk production

C. The period immediately after the birth of the baby and continuing for 6 weeks

D. Separation of the abdominal muscles

E. An immunization to reduce potential harm from Rh antibodies in the future

F. The establishment of a strong emotional attachment during the pregnancy

G. Infection in the breasts

H. Breast tenderness and fullness due to breast milk

I. A hormone responsible for uterine contractions

J. The return of the uterus to the nonpregnant state

FILL IN THE BLANKS

Fill in the blanks with the appropriate word or phrase.

1. After the birth of the baby, the woman will experience vaginal bleeding known as _____.

2. After delivery, the uterus must remain firm and contracted. The term used to refer to the uterus that is not adequately contracted is _____.

3. During the pregnancy, a woman begins to produce a high protein substance in preparation for lactation. This substance is known as _____.

4. After delivery a client begins to shake. This phenomenon is the result of the mother's body temperature being higher than the surrounding environment and is known as the _____.

5. The father of a newborn baby is holding and maintaining eye contact with his son. He voices interest in the care of the child. He is demonstrating

   _____.

6. One week postpartum the new mother appears tired. She states she is weeping for little reason and feels unable to cope. She is experiencing

   _____.

7. While performing an assessment on a postpartum client, the nurse asks the client to sit with legs straight and knees slightly flexed. When the woman's foot was sharply dorsiflexed, she reported pain and tenderness. This is known as a _____.

8. Nursing care must be culturally sensitive. Recently delivered women of Mexican, Asian, and African descent may avoid _____.

MULTIPLE CHOICE

Circle the answer that best completes the following statements.

1. Two hours after delivery, the nurse assesses the postpartum client. The assessment reveals the uterus is not firm. Which of the following actions by the nurse is indicated first?
   1. Assist the client to ambulate to the bathroom.
   2. Administer Pitocin (oxytocin).
   3. Increase the rate of the IV.
   4. Massage the uterus.

2. A fundal assessment on a client who delivered a term infant 5 hours previous reveals the fundus is 1 centimeter above the umbilicus and is deviated to the side. Which of the following interventions should the nurse perform first?
   1. Assist the client to the bathroom.
   2. Do nothing at this time.
   3. Perform a fundal massage.
   4. Attempt to express clots from the uterus.

3. At the fourth postpartum day, which of the following locations of the fundus is considered appropriate?
    1. At the level of the symphysis pubis
    2. At the level of the umbilicus
    3. Four centimeters below the umbilicus
    4. Four centimeters above the symphysis pubis

4. Which of the following reflects the correct sequence of lochia experienced by the postpartal woman?
    1. Lochia alba, lochia serosa, lochia rubra
    2. Lochia rubra, lochia serosa, lochia alba
    3. Lochia serosa, lochia rubra, lochia alba
    4. Lochia rubra, lochia alba, lochia serosa

5. As she is preparing for discharge, a client asks how long it will be until she is fertile. Which of the following statements by the nurse is most correct?
    1. "You may not begin to ovulate for at least 6 months."
    2. "You may be fertile within the next month."
    3. "Breastfeeding will provide you with protection against pregnancy."
    4. "The physician will determine your fertility at your 6-week checkup."

6. The complete blood cell count of a client performed on her first postpartum day reflects a white blood cell count of 20,000/μL. The nurse reviewing this report should take which of the following actions?
    1. Do nothing.
    2. Contact the physician.
    3. Ask the laboratory to reassess the test.
    4. Administer an antibiotic.

7. The day after delivery, the nurse notices a client does not appear to be bonding with her new baby. The client states she thought she would have accomplished more with her life. Which of the responses by the nurse is most therapeutic?
    1. "Do you think you will be able to take your baby home?"
    2. "Tell me how you feel your future accomplishments will be affected."
    3. "Are you open to meeting with a social worker?"
    4. "Do you have help at home until you are feeling better?"

8. While working on the postpartum care unit, you are assigned a mother who is of Asian descent. When you bring her the towels for her to shower, she declines, stating she does not wish to become chilled. Which of the following is the best course of action by the nurse?
    1. Advise her you will contact the physician if she does not take a shower.
    2. Leave the supplies and advise her to let you know if she changes her mind or needs help.
    3. Contact the charge nurse.
    4. Instruct the woman her risk of infection will be greatly increased if she does not take a shower as instructed.

9. You are assigned to provide care to four clients on the postpartum unit. Which of the clients listed below will be most likely to experience the strongest afterpains?
   1. The breastfeeding client who has just had her first child.
   2. The bottle-feeding client who has given birth to her second child.
   3. The bottle-feeding client who has given birth to her first child.
   4. The breastfeeding client who has given birth to her third child.

10. When performing a complete assessment on the postpartum client, the nurse recognizes the fundus is included. Place in order of occurrence the steps the nurse will take when assessing the fundus.
   1. Place one hand on the lower uterine segment.
   2. Ask the woman to void.
   3. Position the woman supine with the knees slightly flexed.
   4. Palpate the abdomen to locate the fundus.

11. During her third postpartum day the client reports she has begun to notice pain and tenderness in her breasts. She asks what can be done to reduce the discomfort being experienced. What recommendations can be made by the nurse to respond to the client's requests? Select all that apply.
   1. Take a warm shower and allow the water to run over her breasts.
   2. Express some breast milk to reduce pain and tenderness.
   3. Apply an ice pack to the breasts.
   4. Wear a support bra or chest binder.

12. The day after delivery, the client reports she has been urinating frequently. She expresses confusion stating she has had little to drink since delivery. Which of the following best explains what is taking place?
   1. The client is experiencing a physiological occurrence known as puerperal diuresis.
   2. The client is simply voiding large amounts in response to the large volume of IV fluids administered during labor.
   3. The frequent voiding is a result of the hormonal changes associated with the end of the pregnancy.
   4. There is no physiological process going on at this time relating to the urinary system.

13. During a visit to the physician's office, a client voices complaints about her abdominal muscle tone. She reports she has been experiencing backaches since her child was born 6 months ago. The physical examination reveals her abdomen is flabby and lacks tone. The physician determines the abdominal muscles separated during the later portion of her pregnancy. Which of the following interventions will be utilized to manage this condition?
   1. Surgical intervention to suction out some of the fat cells.
   2. Surgical intervention to reconnect the torn muscles.
   3. Exercise.
   4. A low carbohydrate diet.

14. When assisting the breastfeeding postpartum client to plan her nutritional needs, which of the following statements should be included in the discussion?
    1. Limit fluid intake.
    2. Increase dietary content by at least 300 calories each day.
    3. Discontinue prenatal vitamins to reduce constipation in the baby.
    4. Begin taking a vitamin K supplement.

15. A breastfeeding postpartum client has complaints of redness, swelling, and tenderness in her left breast. The right breast remains unaffected. Based on your knowledge, which of the following recommendations should be made?
    1. Do nothing.
    2. Discontinue breastfeeding for the next 72 hours to allow the breast to heal.
    3. Reduce breastfeeding in the affected breast and provide formula to the infant to maintain nutritional balance.
    4. Continue breastfeeding and report concerns the physician.

CRITICAL THINKING EXERCISE

Read the case study. Answer the questions, keeping in mind the steps of the nursing process: assessing, diagnosing, planning, implementing, and evaluating.

Two hours after delivery, the client is moved to her room in the postpartum unit. She calls down to the nurse's station and reports feeling "wet." The LPN/LVN responds to the call. The assessment reveals the client's perineal pad is saturated with lochia.

1. After finding the bloody pads, what is the next step the nurse should take?
2. Identify potential limitations of the LPN/LVN regarding care of this client and the scope of practice.
3. What vital sign findings may signal a hemorrhage?
4. Discuss management/treatment intervention that may be employed to care for this client.

Chapter 11

Life Span Growth and Development

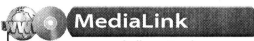

MediaLink

www.prenhall.com/towle

Use the address above to access the free, interactive Companion Website created for this textbook. Get hints, instant feedback to chapter-related NCLEX®-style questions. Link to other interesting sites.

Audio Glossary:

Use the Companion Website, or the CD-ROM disk enclosed with your textbook, to hear the pronunciation of key terms in the chapter.

Throughout a person's life span, they are expected to progress through many changes. The changes experienced include physical changes and cognitive, emotional, and moral development changes. Several theories exist to describe the many changes. These theories of growth and development are guides to be used to evaluate a person's progression through the many stages. Understanding the expected changes and variations will assist the nurse to determine how to approach a client, what the current client's issues may be, and what health promotion teaching may be needed.

MATCHING

Match the term in the left column with the correct definition in the right column.

1. _____ Cephalocaudal   A.   Birth order
2. _____ Cognitive development   B.   Process of increasing physical size
3. _____ Id   C.   Head-to-toe development
4. _____ Percentile   D.   Intellectual ability development
5. _____ Growth   E.   Pleasure-seeking part of personality
6. _____ Proximodistal   F.   Process of maturation
7. _____ Ordinal position   G.   Realistic part of personality
8. _____ Development   H.   Moral system in personality
9. _____ Ego   I.   Center to peripheral development
10. _____ Superego   J.   Population measurement

FILL IN THE BLANKS

Fill in the blanks with the appropriate word or phrase.

1. Sexual maturity can be documented in stages called _____ _____.
2. _____ (farsightedness) and _____ (loss of hearing) are common with age.
3. When the body ages, there is a(n) _____ in the function of organ systems.
4. _____ may affect vision by clouding the lens of the eye.
5. Eye and hair color are examples of _____ characteristics.
6. Development and maturation may be influenced by different expectations based on _____.
7. The child at age 2 begins to use _____ to communicate with others.
8. The last stage of cognitive development, according to Piaget, is _____ _____, when the child gradually completes the development necessary to function as an adult.
9. According to Erikson, the school-age child will be in the _____ _____ _____ stage of psychosocial development.
10. The greatest influence for the teenager is their _____.

MULTIPLE CHOICE

Circle the answer that best completes the following statements.

1. Which statement best reflects overall growth and development?
    1. Changes have a definite starting point.
    2. Changes start complex and develop to simple.
    3. Everyone follows the same pattern.
    4. Development follows a pattern, but is individual in rate.
2. When learning about growth and development, the student understands that:
    1. Infants develop in a head-to-toe pattern.
    2. Infants learn fine motor control before gross motor control.
    3. Infants learn to walk before they have strong balance.
    4. Infants learn to sit up before they are able to control their head.
3. One influence on growth and development that is nonmodifiable is:
    1. Socioeconomic status.
    2. Heredity.
    3. Health risks.
    4. Dietary consumption.
4. A family's cultural customs may influence which of the following areas that affect growth and development? Select all that apply:
    1. Family dynamics
    2. Diet
    3. Activity
    4. Income level

5. The youngest child out of four children may have growth and development influences that:
   1. Are most influenced by cultural beliefs.
   2. May result from what is learned from the older children.
   3. Are a combination of parental and sibling influences.
   4. Are primarily from the parents.

6. Which of the following children would the nurse anticipate to be behind in growth and development?
   1. The child with three older siblings.
   2. The child who lives with his or her mother and stepfather.
   3. The child whose parents are unemployed.
   4. The child who goes to day care twice a week.

7. A child's cognitive development:
   1. Is most influenced by their physical growth.
   2. Thrives on interaction with the environment.
   3. Is easily plotted on a growth chart.
   4. Develops primarily in the first year of life.

8. The psychosocial stage of development for the infant is identified as:
   1. Autonomy versus shame and doubt.
   2. Sensorimotor.
   3. Anal stage.
   4. Trust versus mistrust.

9. The adolescent who says, "I just want to do what all my friends are able to do," is displaying behavior that:
   1. Is suggestive of poor self-esteem.
   2. Is typical of this age of development.
   3. Requires strict rules to follow.
   4. Seems to be behind in typical development for this age.

10. Freud's theory on development is based upon:
    1. Cognitive influences.
    2. Psychosocial influences.
    3. Sexual influences.
    4. Physical influences.

11. Which of the following data would be within the expected range for an infant? Select all that apply.
    1. Birth weight has doubled by 5 months of age.
    2. Birth weight has tripled by 12 months of age.
    3. Has grown 12 inches in length in first year.
    4. Sleeps 20 to 22 hours per day during first 12 months of life.

12. What is the greatest influence on the infant successfully mastering the stage of trust versus mistrust?
    1. Economic status of family
    2. Number of toys they have
    3. Number of siblings
    4. Adult response to physical needs

13. A major accomplishment during the toddler years is:
    1. Learning to walk.
    2. Initiation of toilet training.
    3. Ability to obey rules.
    4. Ability to reason.

14. In which stage of development will children typically move away from believing in fantasy?
    1. Toddler
    2. Preschool
    3. School age
    4. Adolescent

15. A 16-year-old male asks the nurse if he has reached his adult height. The nurse's best response would be:
    1. "You may have since your parents are not very tall."
    2. "You may continue to grow until you are 21 years old."
    3. "Most boys continue to grow until puberty."
    4. "You will need to ask your dad when he stopped growing."

CRITICAL THINKING EXERCISE

Read the case study. Answer the questions, keeping in mind the steps of the nursing process: assessing, diagnosing, planning, implementing, and evaluating.

A $2^1/_2$-year-old is brought to the office by his father for a flu shot. The new graduate nurse walks into the room with the syringe on a tray and asks the child if he will get ready for his shot. The nurse gets frustrated when the child begins to cry and clings to his father. The nurse tries to take the child and put him on the exam table. The child continues to cry, and the nurse eventually leaves the room to get a more experienced nurse. You are the LPN/LVN experienced in working with children. Answer the following questions based on your knowledge of growth and development of a child this age.

1. What stage of development is the child in according to Erikson and Piaget?
2. How can the growth and development level affect the interaction with a child?
3. What are some suggestions based of the growth and development level of this child that the graduate nurse could implement next time?
4. What is the role of the father in this situation?

Chapter 12

Illness Prevention, Health Promotion, and Nutrition in Children

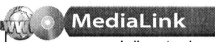

MediaLink

www.prenhall.com/towle

Use the address above to access the free, interactive Companion Website created for this textbook. Get hints, instant feedback to chapter-related NCLEX®-style questions. Link to other interesting sites.

Audio Glossary:

Use the Companion Website, or the CD-ROM disk enclosed with your textbook, to hear the pronunciation of key terms in the chapter.

The nurse's role in caring for children is not just about a focus on disease, but on illness prevention and health promotion. Teaching is one of the primary responsibilities of the nurse each time there is interaction with caregivers of children. Nutritional health promotion teaching is necessary at each stage of development. Understanding the changes that occur during the stages of growth and development will assist the nurse to know what to discuss and why.

MATCHING

Match the term in the left column with the correct definition in the right column.

1. _____ Secondary prevention	A.	Not just the absence of disease
2. _____ Cooperative play	B.	Side-by-side play activity
3. _____ Health	C.	Helps avoid developing health problems
4. _____ Latch-key child	D.	Effective discipline in preschool child
5. _____ Health promotion	E.	Helps to prevent disease complications
6. _____ Associative play	F.	Organized play activities
7. _____ Primary prevention	G.	Unsupervised until parents arrive home
8. _____ "Time-out"	H.	Activities suggested for healthier state
9. _____ Parallel play	I.	Helps detect and treat problems early
10. _____ Tertiary prevention	J.	Sharing together type of play

FILL IN THE BLANKS

Fill in the blanks with the appropriate word or phrase.

1. During the _____ years, health screenings such as tuberculosis, vision, hearing, and blood and urine testing are done.

2. Reducing the level of obesity in children and adolescents to _____ is a goal listed in *Healthy People 2010.*

3. _____ cells are established in childhood.

4. Infants restrained in a car seat should be placed in the _____ _____ when being transported in a car.

5. Infants may show signs of _____ at 4 months.

6. Before 1 year of age, cow's milk is an insufficient source of _____.

7. Motor vehicle crashes, burns, and _____ remain the leading causes of death in _____.

8. The deposit of _____ in the body is five times higher before menarche begins.

9. Adolescents may participate in _____ _____ activities.

10. _____ _____ is a major milestone to begin working on during the toddler years.

MULTIPLE CHOICE

Circle the answer that best completes the following statements.

1. Which of the following activities would be considered tertiary prevention activities? Select all that apply.
    1. Checking school children for lice.
    2. Administering scheduled immunizations to "well" children.
    3. Performing range-of-motion activities to client on bedrest.
    4. Administering antibiotics to prevent spread of tuberculosis.

2. A nurse is teaching school-age children about preventing the spread of germs that may cause disease. Which of the following topics should be included?
    1. Keep soiled tissues on their desk.
    2. Only share a drink if they are not sick.
    3. Cough or sneeze into elbow area.
    4. Wash hands after lunch.

3. Which of the following actions should be documented by the nurse when an immunization is given to a child? Select all that apply.
    1. Size of needle.
    2. Route of administration.
    3. Expiration date of vial or prefilled syringe used.
    4. Lot number on vial or prefilled syringe used.

4. Four parents call the office to ask if their child should still be brought in to receive their scheduled immunization. Which of the following children should still go to the appointment and receive the immunization? Select all that apply.
   1. Child who has had a cold for 3 days with temperature of 99.7°F.
   2. Child who has had a cold for 2 days with temperature of 101.5°F.
   3. Child who is on antibiotics for bilateral ear infections.
   4. Child who is in day care with a child diagnosed with pneumonia.

5. The new graduate nurse is nervous about giving her first immunization injection. Which intervention should the experienced nurse give to help the new nurse?
   1. "Make sure you have the parents help hold the child."
   2. "Be sure to not tell them it will hurt."
   3. "Be honest if they ask if it will hurt."
   4. "Give the child a sticker after if they did not throw a big fit."

6. The parents of a 3-year-old report having trouble disciplining their child. What suggestion by the nurse would be most appropriate?
   1. Give the child two chances to change the behavior.
   2. Use the "time-out" method.
   3. Spank the child if they are about to do something dangerous.
   4. Send the child to their room after the behavior.

7. When discussing growth and development changes to a group of new parents, the nurse discusses the need for play in a child's life. What is the best rationale for the nurse to include this topic?
   1. Play is fun for all involved.
   2. Play will give the parents a chance for a break.
   3. Children learn through play activities.
   4. Some parents may feel guilty about playing too much.

8. When teaching first-time parents about safety for the newborn, the nurse should focus on:
   1. Keeping toys picked up off the floor.
   2. Keeping small objects out of reach.
   3. Placing safety gates at top of stairs.
   4. Safe sleeping measures.

9. Select the toy that is most appropriate for an 8-month-old infant.
   1. Coloring book with crayons.
   2. Play dough.
   3. Puzzles.
   4. Cloth blocks.

10. A parent calls the pediatrician's office to ask if she needs to sterilize her newborn's bottles and nipples. The best response by the nurse would be:
    1. "You only need to sterilize them until the baby is 3 months old."
    2. "Sterilizing is not needed unless you are not sure if your water is safe."
    3. "Sterilizing is needed for all bottles and nipples until the child changes to a cup."
    4. "Sterilizing is needed if you give your baby breast milk in a bottle."

11. What is the correct recommended order of food introduction to an infant?
    1. Meat, vegetables and fruit, then rice cereal.
    2. Rice cereal, meat, then vegetables and fruit.
    3. Fruit and vegetables, rice cereal, then meat.
    4. Rice cereal, vegetables and fruit, then meat.

12. When using the "time-out" method of discipline, children are placed in an area without access for toys or other diversional activities. What is the recommended time a 3-year-old should remain in "time-out"?
    1. 5 minutes
    2. 10 minutes
    3. 20 minutes
    4. 3 minutes

13. A nurse is teaching the parents of a 2-year-old how much the child should be eating at meals. An appropriate measure would be:
    1. Provide 3 types of foods to choose from.
    2. Give 2 tablespoons of each food offered.
    3. Provide a food from each food group.
    4. Give one type of food at a time.

14. What should the primary source of nutrition be for an 18-month-old child?
    1. Cow's milk and table food
    2. Formula and rice cereal
    3. Fruits, vegetables and formula
    4. Cow's milk and rice cereal

15. The nurse is giving teaching to a group of parents regarding child safety. Of the following, which is the best method of promoting safety for children who are old enough to speak and understand words?
    1. Have the child learn to spell their first and last name.
    2. Encourage the family to establish a "password" to identify who the child can trust.
    3. Have the child tell an adult their phone number if lost.
    4. Give the child a cell phone to keep with them at all times.

CRITICAL THINKING EXERCISE

Read the case study. Answer the questions, keeping in mind the steps of the nursing process: assessing, diagnosing, planning, implementing, and evaluating.

A nurse is asked to prepare health promotion teaching to a group of day care providers. The nurse plans the care based on growth and development principles. The focus of the teaching is for the toddler phase of 1 to 3 years of age. The teaching needs to include physical, psychosocial, nutritional, and anticipatory teaching topics.

1. What are the major milestones that occur during the toddler stage of growth and development?

2. What are the safety issues involved with the toddler stage that need to be addressed?

3. What type of play should be expected and encouraged with this age of child?

4. What psychosocial issue is addressed in the toddler phase?

5. What nutritional recommendations should be discussed?

Chapter 13

Adapting Procedures in the Care of Children

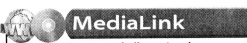
MediaLink
www.prenhall.com/towle

Use the address above to access the free, interactive Companion Website created for this textbook. Get hints, instant feedback to chapter-related NCLEX®-style questions. Link to other interesting sites.

Audio Glossary:
Use the Companion Website, or the CD-ROM disk enclosed with your textbook, to hear the pronunciation of key terms in the chapter.

Each child is at a different stage of physical growth and cognitive/psychosocial development. When assessing and performing procedures on children, the nurse must be familiar with the approach needed as well as actual procedure requirements. This unique focus and the details of procedures that are common in children are addressed in this chapter.

MATCHING

Match the term in the left column with the correct definition in the right column.

1. _____ Residual volume
2. _____ Buccal cavity
3. _____ PEFR meter
4. _____ Vastus lateralis
5. _____ Point of maximal impulse
6. _____ Xiphoid process
7. _____ Preoxygenation
8. _____ Brachial artery
9. _____ Fifth vital sign
10. _____ Left lateral Sims'

A. Site to hear heart best
B. End site of measuring for nasogastric tube
C. Needed before suctioning performed
D. Site for blood pressure in small children
E. Position for enema administration
F. Amount of feeding left in stomach
G. Inside mouth between gum and cheek
H. Pain level
I. Muscle used for injection in infants
J. Used to measure pulmonary function

FILL IN THE BLANKS

Fill in the blanks with the appropriate word or phrase.

1. High levels of oxygen given over a long period of time may damage the
   _____ or _____.

2. When estimating the size needed for an endotracheal tube in a 4-year-old,
   the child's _____ finger should be looked at.

3. When taking the temperature of a child less than 3 years of age, the
   _____ of the _____ should be pulled
   _____ and back.

4. Heart strength is determined by the amount of _____
   exerted with each beat.

5. The BMI is calculated by using the _____ in _____ and
   dividing by the _____ in _____ _____.

6. Head circumference should be measured on any child under _____
   _____ of age.

7. Head circumference is _____ or _____
   centimeters _____ than chest circumference until age _____.

8. When applying a restraint, the child's _____, _____, _____, and
   the _____ are all taken into consideration.

9. In gavage feeding, a tube is inserted through the _____,
   _____, _____ and into the _____.

10. When determining nasogastric tube length, measure from the
    _____ of the _____ to the _____
    of the _____ to the _____ _____.

MULTIPLE CHOICE

Circle the answer that best completes the following statements.

1. Which of the following approach methods would be helpful when preparing
   to do a physical exam on a 3-year-old? Select all that apply.
   1. Allow child to "play" with stethoscope.
   2. Allow parents to remain in room.
   3. Pick child up to place on exam table.
   4. Demonstrate parts of exam on child's doll.

2. A parent is concerned when his child's temperature is found to be one degree
   higher in the emergency department than when it was taken at home. The
   parent reports that the temperature was taken orally at home. What is the
   most probable answer for this?
   1. The parent did not have the thermometer in the mouth for long enough.
   2. The emergency department nurse took the child's temperature rectally.
   3. The child is getting sicker quickly.
   4. The temperature at home was probably taken after the child had a drink.

3. A 6-month-old infant is assessed to find pale skin, respiratory rate of 62, and slow to react to stimulation. What should be the first action of the LPN/LVN?
   1. Administer oxygen at 6 liters per nasal cannula.
   2. Call a "code."
   3. Monitor for 30 minutes and reassess.
   4. Report findings to RN or physician.

4. The nurse is preparing to measure the blood pressure of a 9-month-old infant. Which of the following sites would be appropriate to use with this age of child? Select all that apply.
   1. Upper thigh
   2. Calf
   3. Upper arm
   4. Forearm

5. The newly graduated LPN/LVN is in orientation. He is asked to describe the best plan for measuring a pulse rate on a 4-month-old infant. Which of the following responses is most accurate?
   1. "I will just use the radial site because most babies are very active."
   2. "I need to count the pulse rate for 15 seconds and multiply by four for the total."
   3. "I need to auscultate for a full minute at the apex of the heart."
   4. "I will need to palpate the brachial artery for 1 full minute."

6. The new graduate is having difficulty assessing respiratory rates on younger children. The preceptor nurse offers assistance in assessing the rate on an 8-month-old infant. Which rationale would be given for how to assess the rate on this age of child?
   1. "Children are difficult to count respiratory rates on. Just try the best you can for at least 1 full minute."
   2. "You need to watch the abdomen on a child this age rise and fall to get an accurate count as young children breathe from their diaphragm."
   3. "You can just put your hand on their chest to count the rate."
   4. "Place them on their abdomen and then count the rate."

7. The nurse is concerned because she is not able to determine when the last sound is heard during blood pressure measurement of a 6-year-old child. The most likely reason for this is:
   1. An electrical measurement needs to be taken.
   2. The diastolic pressure is noted as a muffling, not disappearance of sound in children less than 12 years of age.
   3. Another measurement site should be used.
   4. A special stethoscope should be used.

8. Assessing pain in children is part of a routine assessment. What factor might make the assessment of this area more challenging in children?
   1. The child is nonverbal.
   2. The parents are not present.
   3. The child speaks another language.
   4. The child has attention deficit disorder.

9. When determining issues related to a child's weight, what tool would be most helpful to use in children age 2 through adolescence?
   1. Weight of parents
   2. Child's weight
   3. BMI for age
   4. Child's eating habit

10. A 2-year-old child is brought to a clinic for a well-child check. What measurements will be done as initial, routine screening? Select all that apply.
    1. Height
    2. Weight
    3. Head circumference
    4. Blood lead level

11. A newborn infant is being fed through nasogastric tube feedings of expressed breast milk from the mother. Which of the following assessment parameters is indicated prior to each feeding?
    1. Abdominal girth
    2. Chest circumference
    3. Number of wet diapers since last feeding
    4. Residual volume of feeding in stomach

12. When preparing to place a nasogastric tube for feeding, how should the length of insertion be determined?
    1. Based on the child's age
    2. In conjunction with the chest circumference
    3. By measuring from the nose to ear to xiphoid process
    4. Based on the length of the child

13. A child is in need of an enema for assistance with bowel evacuation. Once the physician writes the order, the nurse reviews it. Which type of fluid should the nurse expect to see written for use as an enema in a child?
    1. Water
    2. Hypotonic solution
    3. Isotonic solution
    4. Hypertonic solution

14. An infant is congested and has a respiratory illness. Which of the following would the nurse expect to be used in an infant with this illness?
    1. Oxygen by mask
    2. Nasogastric suctioning
    3. Endotracheal suctioning
    4. Bulb syringe

15. When preparing to suction the trachea of a 2-year-old, what is the maximum amount of time that suction should be applied to the catheter during the removal process?
    1. 5 seconds
    2. 5 to 10 seconds
    3. 10 seconds
    4. 15 seconds

Read the case study. Answer the questions, keeping in mind the steps of the nursing process: assessing, diagnosing, planning, implementing, and evaluating.

A 3-year-old child is brought into the emergency department with a fever of unknown origin. The fever has been up to 103°F for the past 24 hours. The parents report the child will not eat, has had trouble sleeping, and has hardly urinated at all. The child is admitted to the pediatric unit after the initial exam and diagnostic tests are completed.

1. What are the possible diagnostic tests that would be indicated for this diagnosis and in what order?

2. What special considerations would be taken by the emergency department nurse with this child?

3. What sites and/or methods would be used to measure vital signs?

4. When the child needs to have additional blood tests and the intravenous line restarted, what special considerations would be used?

Chapter 14

Care of the Hospitalized or Chronically Ill Child

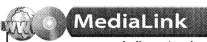

MediaLink
www.prenhall.com/towle

Use the address above to access the free, interactive Companion Website created for this textbook. Get hints, instant feedback to chapter-related NCLEX®-style questions. Link to other interesting sites.

Audio Glossary:

Use the Companion Website, or the CD-ROM disk enclosed with your textbook, to hear the pronunciation of key terms in the chapter.

Children and their families require special attention when the child is hospitalized or has a chronic illness. Hospitalizations and diagnoses of a chronic illness are usually a shock to a child and family. Nurses have the opportunity to ensure the process and care is delivered in a timely manner, is appropriate to the child's age, and is performed correctly. By reviewing concepts and plans of care for these situations, the nurse can be better prepared to provide high-quality, caring interventions to the child and family.

MATCHING

Match the term in the left column with the correct definition in the right column.

1. _____ Therapeutic play	A.	Medication-induced altered consciousness
2. _____ First separation stage	B.	Rapid onset with severe symptoms
3. _____ Illness	C.	Despair
4. _____ Second separation stage	D.	Needs rehabilitation
5. _____ Chronic	E.	Plans activities for child in hospital
6. _____ Third stage of separation	F.	State of disease or sickness
7. _____ Conscious sedation	G.	Detachment
8. _____ Acute	H.	Health-related interaction with a child
9. _____ Child life specialist	I.	Protest
10. _____ Legg-Calvé-Perthes disease	J.	Long-lasting and slow to progress

FILL IN THE BLANKS

Fill in the blanks with the appropriate word or phrase.

1. Common postoperative exercises include _____ _____, coughing and use of an _____ _____.

2. An incentive spirometer is used to promote _____ _____.

3. The administration of intravenous medication to induce an altered level of consciousness is _____ _____.

4. The time to start preparing for discharge is during _____.

5. After physiological needs are met, the priority of care for a hospitalized child is to make sure they feel _____ and _____.

6. _____ _____ can help children feel more comfortable with medical equipment.

7. Children with a chronic illness inherited from their parents are known to have a _____ _____.

8. A chronic disorder that the child was born with is known as a _____ _____.

9. Parents of children with chronic illnesses are very _____.

10. An interdisciplinary plan that addresses the special needs of a specific student is known as what type of plan: _____ _____ _____.

MULTIPLE CHOICE

Circle the answer that best completes the following statements.

1. The nurse needs to understand that families and children who are hospitalized:
   1. Are usually able to catch up on their sleep while in the hospital.
   2. Are usually very stressed about being in the hospital.
   3. Generally like to be left alone while in the hospital.
   4. Are resentful of needing the nurse for so many things.

2. In order to care for the child to the highest level possible, the nurse needs to understand several issues. Select all that apply.
   1. Family composition
   2. Vacation plans
   3. Cultural beliefs
   4. Religious beliefs

3. A 12-year-old child is in the hospital with a fractured femur. After 5 days, the physician decides that 5 to 10 more days of hospitalization is needed. What should the nurse plan to address with the child and the family based on this information?
   1. The child will get a roommate at some point.
   2. The child will need to obtain schoolwork to do while being hospitalized.
   3. The family will need financial counseling.
   4. The parents need to be able to go home and sleep.

4. A 5-year-old child has been scheduled for a tonsillectomy. Which of the following interventions would be most appropriate for the child and family?
   1. Have a child who has had the surgery talk to this child.
   2. Provide drawings of tonsils out of a medical textbook.
   3. Provide a tour of the hospital prior to surgery.
   4. Send a pamphlet in the mail about the surgery.

5. An 18-month-old child is hospitalized for pneumonia. The parents need to go home to care for the other four siblings. Which of the following behaviors would be expected by the child over the next day once the parents leave? Select all that apply.
   1. Crying
   2. Laying quietly in crib
   3. Disinterest in favorite toys
   4. Disinterest in parents when they return

6. A 10-month-old child has been hospitalized for 10 days for failure to thrive. When the nurse enters the room for the morning assessment, the child smiles and holds out her arms to the nurse to be held. The nurse understands that this child is in which stage of separation anxiety?
   1. Denial
   2. Despair
   3. Protest
   4. Detachment

7. The parents of a 3-year-old child hospitalized with a gastrointestinal disorder leave several times a day. They wait until the child is playing with toys and then "sneak out." This behavior can cause what reaction in the child?
   1. The child will continue to play if they are favorite toys.
   2. The child will want the nurse to stay in the room to play.
   3. The child will lose trust in the parents.
   4. The child will cry until the parents return.

8. A 2-year-old child is in need of an intramuscular injection. The 4-year-old brother begins to cry and says, "It is really going to hurt him!" The 2-year-old begins to cry. What reaction by the nurse would be the most appropriate in this situation?
   1. Tell the sibling that he needs to leave the room.
   2. Ask the parents to tell the 2-year-old that it will not hurt.
   3. Ask another nurse that the child is not familiar with to go in to give the injection.
   4. Explain briefly what will happen and that it will hurt for "just a little bit."

9. The hospitalized 4-year-old is upset after the admission process is complete. The mother asks him why he is so upset. He cries and says that he knows he got sick because he was mean to his younger sibling. The nurse can assist the mother in this situation by:
   1. Having her bring the sibling in so the 4-year-old can apologize.
   2. Explaining that this type of thinking is typical of this age group.
   3. Asking the physician for a psychological consult.
   4. Encouraging the mother to just ignore this behavior and it will go away.

10. The school-age child would most likely be interested in assisting with which of the following tasks while in the hospital for a respiratory illness? Select all that apply.
    1. Writing down how much they drink.
    2. Performing their Triflow exercises during each cartoon commercial.
    3. Holding the tape during their intravenous line insertion.
    4. Assisting with changing the bed linens.

11. The mother of a 15-year-old who is hospitalized with abdominal pain for 4 days asks the nurse what she can do to get her child in better spirits. The best response by the nurse would be to:
    1. Request a psychological referral from the physician.
    2. Ask a hospital clergy member to visit.
    3. Suggest that friends be allowed to visit for an hour in the afternoon.
    4. Buy the child a new book.

12. A 7-year-old child is being prepared for surgery. The child has never had surgery before and is very nervous. The nurse can suggest which intervention that would be best to assist in decreasing the child's anxiety?
    1. Give the child a surgical mask to try on.
    2. Show the child a picture of the recovery room.
    3. Administer sedative medication.
    4. Tell the child about other children who have had surgery.

13. After teaching an 8-year-old child about her surgery to have an appendectomy, which response by the child would demonstrate effective preoperative teaching by the nurse?
    1. The child applies a bandage to her stuffed animal at the site of where an appendix would be located.
    2. The child cries when anyone mentions the surgery.
    3. The child becomes quiet and just wants to sleep.
    4. The child tells a parent that she does not want to do the deep breathing after surgery.

14. The parents of a 12-year-old postoperative male are concerned about the physician's order to use a PCA (patient-controlled analgesia) pump on their son. The father states, "We think he will overdose and push the button too many times because he has attention deficit disorder." The nurse's teaching in response to this comment should focus on:
    1. How much of a problem the child's attention deficit issue causes with activities.
    2. The safety features set in the pump and by the programming nurses.
    3. What to do if an overdose occurs.
    4. Discussing the maximum amount the nurse thinks the child should use.

15. A primary safety feature of the process in initiating and administering medication by PCA (patient controlled analgesia) is:
    1. It can only be used on children who weigh more than 100 pounds.
    2. It can only be used postoperative for simple surgeries.
    3. Two licensed nurses double-check all pump entries and orders.
    4. The child is kept on bedrest while the pump is in use.

CRITICAL THINKING EXERCISE

Read the case study. Answer the questions, keeping in mind the steps of the nursing process: assessing, diagnosing, planning, implementing, and evaluating.

An 8-year-old child is being admitted to the pediatric unit after being diagnosed with acute appendicitis. The surgeon has scheduled the child for surgery the following morning. The child is at the appropriate growth and developmental levels. The nurse caring for the child preoperatively is just learning about children with surgical needs.

1. What tools appropriate for this age of child can the nurse use to educate the child about the procedure?
2. What are the specific preoperative teaching needs?
3. What are some specific postoperative needs?
4. What unique ideas might be implemented to meet the postoperative needs?
5. What is the role of the parent in the care of this child?

Chapter 15

Care of the Child with Fluid, Electrolyte, and Acid-Base Disorders

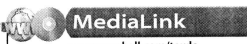

www.prenhall.com/towle

Use the address above to access the free, interactive Companion Website created for this textbook. Get hints, instant feedback to chapter-related NCLEX®-style questions. Link to other interesting sites.

Audio Glossary:

Use the Companion Website, or the CD-ROM disk enclosed with your textbook, to hear the pronunciation of key terms in the chapter.

Subtle changes in fluid levels can have a tremendous impact on a child's health. Illness, disease, and medications can affect the fluid, electrolyte, and acid-base balance. Close monitoring of a child's fluid status is required to detect any problems at the earliest stage. The nurse is responsible for this close monitoring and assessment.

MATCHING

Match the term in the left column with the correct dfinition in the right column.

1. _____ Dehydration	A.	High hydrogen ions
2. _____ ABG	B.	Solutes in body fluid
3. _____ Hyperkalemia	C.	Decreased hydrogen ions
4. _____ Respiratory alkalosis	D.	Fluid volume deficit
5. _____ Homeostasis	E.	Rapid and deep respirations
6. _____ Acidosis	F.	Most common type of dehydration
7. _____ Kussmaul	G.	Acid-base status measurement
8. _____ Electrolytes	H.	Balance of fluid and electrolytes
9. _____ Alkalosis	I.	Increased potassium blood level
10. _____ Isotonic	J.	Low carbon dioxide level

FILL IN THE BLANKS

Fill in the blanks with the appropriate word or phrase.

1. A child's weight is _____% water.

2. An infant's weight is _____% water.

3. A newborn's weight is _____% water.

4. _____ _____ is the best way to monitor fluid balance.

5. _____ is the value used to calculate fluid requirements in children.

6. When weighing a diaper, one _____ equals _____ milliliter of fluid.

7. In the pediatric population, nearly _____% are related to some type of dehydration.

8. The _____ of body _____ lost will determine the level of dehydration.

9. Edema is usually _____ in infants and _____ in children.

10. _____ can progress to pulmonary edema.

MULTIPLE CHOICE

Circle the answer that best completes the following statements.

1. Which of the following intravenous fluids would be most appropriate for a client with burns?
   1. D 5 0.9% normal saline
   2. Normal saline
   3. Lactated Ringer's
   4. D 5 water

2. When teaching a client about foods that can increase potassium, what food choices should be encouraged?
   1. Meats such as chicken and pork
   2. Fruits such as bananas and oranges
   3. Vegetables such as corn and green beans
   4. Carbohydrates such as bagels and bread

3. An experienced nurse is preparing to teach a new nurse who is on orientation about blood gas interpretation (ABGs). What will be the first step that the nurse will be instructed to do with the data from the ABG?
   1. Review the $PaCO_2$
   2. Review the HCO_3
   3. Review the pH
   4. Review the oxygen saturation

4. A school nurse is preparing an educational session with parents on self-asphyxiation. One of the common signs to be noted in the child participating in this activity would be:
   1. High-pitched voice, even in males.
   2. Bruising on the upper forehead.
   3. Petechiae on the face.
   4. Circumoral cyanosis.

5. Which of the following types of medications would alert the nurse to investigate further when a child has a fluid and electrolyte problem? Select all that apply.
   1. Antibiotics
   2. Steroids
   3. Diuretics
   4. Pain medications

6. A parent calls the pediatrician's office seeking advice on what to do for her child who has been vomiting for the past 6 hours. After doing a brief phone assessment, the nurse determines that the child can be managed at home for the time being. What advice would the nurse most likely suggest as an intervention related to fluid status?
   1. Have the mother give an antiemetic.
   2. Have the mother hold all fluids until the vomiting stops for 4 hours.
   3. Encourage small amounts of oral fluids every 10 minutes.
   4. Try to get the child to sleep for a while.

7. What are the values that the nurse will review when ABG results are available? Select all that apply.
   1. Lead level
   2. Carbon dioxide
   3. pH
   4. Bicarbonate

8. In a child who has a respiratory illness, such as respiratory acidosis, what is the nurse's priority in caring for this child?
   1. Monitoring vital signs
   2. Monitoring oxygen level
   3. Monitoring level of consciousness
   4. Maintaining a patent airway

9. A child who has been vomiting for the past 24 hours is brought into the emergency department. The nurse starts to review in their head what type of situation will be anticipated for this child to make a diagnosis. Based on the presenting symptom, what would the nurse anticipate will be discovered?
   1. Respiratory alkalosis
   2. Metabolic alkalosis
   3. Respiratory acidosis
   4. Metabolic acidosis

10. A 12-year-old child is admitted with metabolic acidosis. The child has a history of diabetes and poor nutritional habits. What will the nurse expect the lab results to indicate?
   1. Kussmaul respiratory status
   2. Cardiac dysrhythmias
   3. Ketoacidosis
   4. Hyponatremia

11. When discussing health issues with a group of high school children, the nurse is asked why people are told to breathe into a paper bag at times. The best response by the nurse would be:
    1. "You should never do that. It may cause you to have breathing difficulty."
    2. "When you feel dizzy and are starting to get anxious and afraid."
    3. "When you are sleepy."
    4. "When you are getting ready to go swimming."

12. When assessing a client who is diagnosed as having respiratory acidosis, the nurse would expect to find which of the following?
    1. Low blood pressure
    2. Rapid respiratory rate
    3. Low temperature
    4. High pain level

13. Evaluate the following ABG results and determine the problem:
    pH 7. 34, $PaCO_2$ 48, HCO_3 23.
    1. Metabolic alkalosis
    2. Metabolic acidosis
    3. Respiratory alkalosis
    4. Respiratory acidosis

14. A nurse is assessing a child who has had a gastrointestinal virus for 3 days. The child has been vomiting and has had severe diarrhea. In order to determine fluid status before any labs are drawn, what can the nurse assess for? Select all that apply.
    1. Skin turgor
    2. Skin color
    3. Mucous membrane color and moisture level
    4. Height

15. An infant is given a diagnosis of failure to thrive. The nurse is assessing the infant for the first time. What assessment data would be useful to gather in this 8-month-old infant to determine fluid status quickly?
    1. Urine specific gravity
    2. Body mass index
    3. Fontanel level
    4. ABGs

CRITICAL THINKING EXERCISE

Read the case study. Answer the questions, keeping in mind the steps of the nursing process: assessing, diagnosing, planning, implementing, and evaluating.

An infant is brought to the physician's office with weight loss. The infant is 8 months old and has lost 2 pounds in the past month. The mother reports that the father of the baby just lost his job. She is unable to give a detailed account of the volume and frequency of the infant's feedings.

1. What are the components of the nursing assessment that focus on the chief complaint?
2. What other symptoms would the nurse anticipate finding?
3. What acid-base disorder might this infant have?
4. What are two potential nursing diagnoses for this situation related to fluid status or acid-base imbalance?

Chapter 16

Care of the Child with Neurological and Sensory Disorders

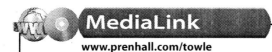

www.prenhall.com/towle

Use the address above to access the free, interactive Companion Website created for this textbook. Get hints, instant feedback to chapter-related NCLEX®-style questions. Link to other interesting sites.

Audio Glossary:

Use the Companion Website, or the CD-ROM disk enclosed with your textbook, to hear the pronunciation of key terms in the chapter.

The child with a neurological disorder may present a challenge for assessment. The nurse must be able to distinguish typical behavior from pathological behavior. Assessing the different age groups neurologically can be difficult. This chapter discusses some of the common childhood medical situations, including otitis media, or the common ear infection.

MATCHING

Match the term in the left column with the correct definition in the right column.

1. _____ Glasgow Coma Scale   A.   Chronic seizure disorder

2. _____ Meningocele   B.   Transports nutrients and removes waste

3. _____ Parasympathetic   C.   Fifth vital sign

4. _____ Status epilepticus   D.   Spinal cord and meninges herniation

5. _____ CSF   E.   Assists body in stressful situation

6. _____ Epilepsy   F.   Precedes a seizure

7. _____ Pain   G.   Herniation of the meninges

8. _____ Myelomeningocele   H.   Nervous system that controls nonstressful situations

9. _____ Aura   I.   Level of consciousness score

10. _____ Sympathetic   J.   Continuous seizure

FILL IN THE BLANKS

Fill in the blanks with the appropriate word or phrase.

1. A patch should be removed for _____ hours each day when worn for amblyopia.

2. The _____ _____ of the young child is shorter and wider than that of the older child. This shape increases the risk of _____ _____.

3. _____ may be reported and is an unusual ringing in the ears.

4. _____ is a common learning disability that has a neurological basis.

5. A child who is unable to coordinate the eye muscles is known to have _____.

6. Problems with visual acuity may be _____ (farsightedness) or _____ (nearsightedness).

7. Down syndrome, also known as _____ _____, is caused by an extra _____.

8. The majority of cases of meningitis occur in children _____ age _____.

9. _____ meningitis is the more serious of the two types.

10. The disorder that affects motor function and posture is known as _____ _____.

MULTIPLE CHOICE

Circle the answer that best completes the following statements.

1. A 7-month-old infant is brought to the office for a well-child check. As the nurse is assessing the fontanel, the father asks why the nurse is feeling the top of the baby's head. The best response by the nurse would be:
   1. "To check for any signs of injury."
   2. "To make sure the soft spot is closed."
   3. "The baby's soft spot, or fontanel, is checked because it usually does not close until about 2 years of age."
   4. "To see how the baby reacts when their head is touched."

2. A child was born with a brain injury. The child is now 4 months old and is in the emergency department after having a seizure at home. What are some early signs of increased intracranial pressure? Select all that apply.
   1. High-pitched crying
   2. Sunken fontanel
   3. Dilated scalp veins
   4. Vomiting

3. While in the neuro-intensive care unit, the nurse assesses the client for which late signs of increased intracranial pressure? Select all that apply.
   1. Tachycardia
   2. Bradycardia
   3. Increased blood pressure
   4. Decreased blood pressure

4. The nurse is providing teaching to a woman in the physician's office. She has just found out that she is pregnant. What teaching will the nurse provide about spina bifida?
   1. The mother should have an early sonogram if this is suspected.
   2. The mother should make sure to take a prenatal vitamin that contains folic acid.
   3. The mother should eat foods high in acid in the last trimester.
   4. The mother should have her blood pressure taken weekly.

5. A child is born with a myelomeningocele. The parents are very upset and asking questions about the extent of the neurological damage. The nurse knows that the child may have (select all that apply):
   1. Seizures
   2. Flaccid paralysis
   3. Sensory deficits
   4. Bowel and bladder incontinence

6. A child with a myelomeningocele is suspected of having hydrocephalus. The nurse will focus on looking for what classic sign of this?
   1. High-pitched cry
   2. Low blood pressure
   3. Enlarged upper head circumference
   4. Dilated pupils

7. A shunt has been placed in an 8-month-old child with hydrocephalus. The child is in the recovery room. The nurse notes the head of the child's bed is up 30 degrees. The nurse should:
   1. Leave the child in this position until taking to the room.
   2. Pick the child up to keep them from crying.
   3. Lower the head of the bed to keep the child flat.
   4. Raise the head of the bed up to 45 degrees.

8. The parents of a child who has been diagnosed with amyotrophic lateral sclerosis are asking questions related to the child's prognosis. The nurse understands that:
   1. The child can only recover with a bone marrow transplant.
   2. The child will probably experience severe seizures as they progress.
   3. The child will be able to survive if they remain physically active.
   4. The usual cause of death is respiratory failure.

9. A 6-month-old child is brought to the emergency department after a seizure at day care. What data would indicate that the child has had a febrile seizure?
   1. The child has had a low-grade fever for 3 days.
   2. The child's temperature was fine in the morning, but rose to 102 degrees by lunchtime.
   3. The child received acetaminophen (Tylenol) just prior to the seizure.
   4. The child had been diagnosed with an ear infection the week before.

10. When teaching the parents of a child who had a febrile seizure, the nurse discusses which intervention that is no longer recommended?
    1. Administering acetaminophen (Tylenol)
    2. Unwrapping the child from multiple blankets
    3. Taking the child to the emergency department if the child also has a fever with the seizure
    4. Using rubbing alcohol baths to decrease fever

11. A 2-year-old is noted to be sleepy and unable to sit up after the child's seizure has stopped. The parents are concerned that this indicates brain damage has occurred. The nurse's response would include:
    1. Reassurance that seizures do not cause brain damage.
    2. Teaching that this is common in the postictal stage related to seizures.
    3. Teaching that further testing will need to be done based on the responses after the seizure.
    4. Remaining neutral in all responses related to the child's prognosis.

12. A nursing instructor is reviewing with her students the steps to be taken if a child has a seizure. What is the first step one would take?
    1. Insert an oral airway.
    2. Place the child on a cardiac monitor.
    3. Turn the child on his or her side.
    4. Apply oxygen immediately.

13. A suspected diagnosis of meningitis has been made. Which one of the following signs and symptoms would be indicative of meningococcal meningitis?
    1. Seizures
    2. Slurred speech
    3. Petechiae rash
    4. Large pupils

14. The diagnosis of meningitis has been confirmed in a 3-year-old child. Before entering the child's room to provide care, the nurse must put on what type of protective equipment?
    1. None needed with this diagnosis
    2. Mask and gloves
    3. Gown and gloves
    4. Gown, mask, and gloves

15. The nurse is providing teaching to a group of parents who have school-age children. When teaching about medications, what should the nurse discuss about medicating children for fevers?
    1. No medication should be given until it is known if the child has a febrile seizure.
    2. Only children over the age of 2 can be medicated for fevers.
    3. It is best to just wait out the fever and give no medication.
    4. A child should not be given aspirin for pain or fever relief.

CRITICAL THINKING EXERCISE

Read the case study. Answer the questions, keeping in mind the steps of the nursing process: assessing, diagnosing, planning, implementing, and evaluating.

A 5-month-old infant and his 3-year-old sibling are being seen in the pediatrician's office for a sick visit. Both children have had a runny nose and low-grade fever for the past 2 days. The mother is concerned that they might have ear infections based on their behaviors.

1. What is the medial term for an ear infection?
2. Why are younger children more prone to this type of infection?
3. What are the signs and symptoms of an ear infection in an infant and then in a verbal child?
4. What is a possible treatment for a child with a recurrent ear infection?
5. What is the care of the child who is treated surgically for a chronic ear infection?

Chapter 17

Care of the Child with Musculoskeletal Disorders

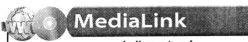

www.prenhall.com/towle

Use the address above to access the free, interactive Companion Website created for this textbook. Get hints, instant feedback to chapter-related NCLEX®-style questions. Link to other interesting sites.

Audio Glossary:

Use the Companion Website, or the CD-ROM disk enclosed with your textbook, to hear the pronunciation of key terms in the chapter.

Musculoskeletal disorders are common to pediatric care. There are problems that may be evident at birth and some that are not noticeable until adolescence. The nurse must be familiar with the basic assessment and care of the child with common musculoskeletal issues. Management of these disorders will require specific knowledge of anatomy and physiology. The nursing process can guide the nurse with this care.

MATCHING

Match the term in the left column with the correct definition in the right column.

1. _____ Ortolani-Barlow
2. _____ Greenstick
3. _____ Torticollis
4. _____ Knock knees
5. _____ Closed reduction
6. _____ Epiphyseal plate
7. _____ Scoliosis
8. _____ Kyphosis
9. _____ Bowed legs
10. _____ Open reduction

A. Buckling
B. Surgical adjustment
C. Genu varum
D. S-curvature
E. Genu valgum
F. Hip click
G. Lumbar curvature
H. Manual adjustment
I. Growth plate
J. Wry neck

FILL IN THE BLANKS

Fill in the blanks with the appropriate word or phrase.

1. The most common cause of osteomyelitis in children is _____ _____.

2. Bone tumors are usually found in the _____ _____, _____ _____ or _____ _____.

3. An elevated _____ _____ _____ may be seen in osteosarcoma.

4. Children age _____ to _____ have the highest incidence of Ewing's sarcoma.

5. Treatment of Ewing's sarcoma includes _____ to reduce the size of the tumor.

6. A priority nursing role in caring for children with musculoskeletal disorders is to promote _____.

7. Children in traction need attention for their _____ needs as well as physical needs.

8. Torticollis is caused by the rotation of the _____ _____.

9. _____ _____ requires surgery to insert a rod and fuse the spine.

10. The discomfort of muscles stretching and bones growing is known as _____ _____.

MULTIPLE CHOICE

Circle the answer that best completes the following statements.

1. A child is diagnosed with a "greenstick" fracture of the radius of the right arm. When talking with the parents, the nurse knows that the teaching with this fracture has been effective based on which comment from one of the parents?
   1. "We know this means our child may have an underlying bone disease."
   2. "Our child must be really strong to sustain a fracture of this type."
   3. "A child's bones are not as solid as an adult's are."
   4. "We understand that further investigation into this type of fracture is necessary."

2. The new nursery nurse has just learned how to do a newborn assessment. The nurse notices some variances when assessing the infant's legs and hips. The experienced nurse points out key features that are present with developmental hip dysplasia. These points would include (select all that apply):
   1. Curvature of the spine
   2. Shortening of the femur
   3. Limited abduction of the affected side
   4. Uneven gluteal folds

3. The parents of an infant with developmental hip dysplasia are in need of further teaching based on which comment to the nurse?
   1. "We are glad that this will just require medication to fix."
   2. "We plan to keep the harness on except during a bath."
   3. "It may take over 3 months for this to be fixed."
   4. "The ligaments can be trained and strengthened to hold the hip in place."

4. Which of the following infants would be most likely to have Duchenne's muscular dystrophy?
   1. Twin girls
   2. Premature girl
   3. Full-term male
   4. Full-term female

5. The nurse notices that a 4-year-old male who is in the office for a well-child check uses his upper arms to move from a sitting position on the floor to a standing position. What is this indicative of?
   1. A fractured femur
   2. Developmental hip dysplasia
   3. Gowers' maneuver
   4. Laziness

6. Which of the following might be delayed in a child who has Duchenne's muscular dystrophy?
   1. Talking
   2. Hearing
   3. Reading
   4. Walking

7. Which of the following may be present at the later stages of Duchenne's muscular dystrophy? Select all that apply.
   1. Malnutrition
   2. Enlarged calf muscles
   3. Scoliosis
   4. Respiratory difficulty

8. Select the diet that would be most appropriate for the nurse to teach to parents of a child with muscular dystrophy.
   1. High calorie, low protein, low fiber
   2. High calorie, high protein, low fiber
   3. Low calorie, high protein, high fiber
   4. Low calorie, high protein, low fiber

9. Primary treatment for a 12-year-old child with Osgood-Schlatter disease would include:
   1. Rest.
   2. Surgery.
   3. Medication.
   4. Physical therapy.

10. Legg-Calvé-Perthes disease is characterized by what outcome?
    1. Amputation of the affected leg.
    2. A new femoral head will form after 3 years.
    3. A permanent limp.
    4. Inability to run.

11. A 13-year-old girl is diagnosed with moderate scoliosis. She is crying in her room. The nurse understands that she would be most upset about:
    1. Having surgery to correct the curvature.
    2. Wearing a brace for 23 hours a day.
    3. Being unable to participate in sports.
    4. Having a permanent disability.

12. One permanent effect of surgical intervention to correct a case of severe scoliosis would include:
    1. Being unable to bend forward.
    2. Having to wear a brace for life.
    3. Needing crutches to walk.
    4. Being confined to a wheelchair.

13. While participating in a cheerleading clinic, an 11-year-old girl sprains her ankle. The immediate treatment of this type of injury would include (select all that apply):
    1. Steroid injections.
    2. Application of ice.
    3. Elevation of injured leg.
    4. Resting of leg for 24–36 hours.

14. A child has had surgery to repair a fractured femur. The nurse is assessing the child postoperatively. Which of the following assessment findings would cause the nurse to notify the physician?
    1. Palpable pedal pulse.
    2. Decreased sensation.
    3. Pain relief with intravenous medication.
    4. Able to slowly move leg and foot.

15. The most difficult part of caring for a child in skeletal traction includes:
    1. Keeping the pin sites clean.
    2. Keeping the child mediated for pain.
    3. Keeping the child in alignment.
    4. Keeping the weights at the end of the bed.

CRITICAL THINKING EXERCISE

Read the case study. Answer the questions, keeping in mind the steps of the nursing process: assessing, diagnosing, planning, implementing, and evaluating.

A 2-year-old child is brought to the emergency department with a fractured right femur. The parents report that the child was fine, but just kept crying when trying to stand up. The child requires surgery to repair the fracture. Skeletal traction will be necessary. The child does not smile or talk to the parents.

1. What are the needs of this child?
2. What will happen to the child after the traction time is complete?
3. What would be an area to assess in further detail related to this scenario?
4. What will be a primary nursing diagnosis related to this scenario?

Chapter 18

Care of the Child with Respiratory Disorders

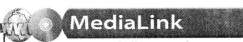

www.prenhall.com/towle

Use the address above to access the free, interactive Companion Website created for this textbook. Get hints, instant feedback to chapter-related NCLEX®-style questions. Link to other interesting sites.

Audio Glossary:

Use the Companion Website, or the CD-ROM disk enclosed with your textbook, to hear the pronunciation of key terms in the chapter.

Caring for a child with a respiratory disorder requires detailed assessment skills. Being able to detect a subtle change can mean avoidance of an emergency situation. Because of the chronic nature of many childhood respiratory illnesses such as asthma and cystic fibrosis, the nurse must be knowledgeable enough about the common respiratory disorders during childhood to provide teaching to a child and his or her caregivers.

MATCHING

Match the term in the left column with the correct definition in the right column.

1. _____ Orthopnea
2. _____ Nasopharyngitis
3. _____ Epistaxis
4. _____ Epiglottitis
5. _____ Dyspnea
6. _____ Tripod position
7. _____ Apnea
8. _____ Tonsillectomy
9. _____ Dysphagia
10. _____ Stridor

A. Sitting upright and leaning forward
B. Surgical removal of palatine tonsils
C. Increased breathing while sitting
D. Absence of breathing
E. Difficulty swallowing
F. High-pitched inspiratory sound
G. Bacterial infection
H. Nasal bleeding
I. Difficulty breathing
J. "Common cold"

FILL IN THE BLANKS

Fill in the blanks with the appropriate word or phrase.

1. The _____ _____ _____ is diagnostic for cystic fibrosis.

2. _____ should only be used with bacterial infections.

3. Cystic fibrosis is a(n) _____ _____ disorder that affects children.

4. The two major body systems affected in cystic fibrosis are the _____ and _____ systems.

5. _____, or air in the chest cavity, can result from trauma.

6. The home should be kept _____ for those children with asthma or other chronic respiratory illnesses.

7. A medical emergency that develops during severe respiratory distress and bronchospasms that does not respond to medications is known as _____ _____.

8. _____ is the leading cause of death in infants between _____ month and _____ year of age.

9. A diagnosis of bronchopulmonary dysplasia (BPD) is based on a _____ _____.

10. _____ _____ _____ _____ is commonly seen in _____ infants.

MULTIPLE CHOICE

Circle the answer that best completes the following statements.

1. The student nurse asks why children and not many adults have tonsillectomies. The nurse's best rationale for this would be:
    1. Physicians find it easier to just have them removed as children.
    2. Adults do not ever need their tonsils removed.
    3. Tonsil tissue atrophies in midadolescence.
    4. Children tend to forget about their surgeries more quickly.

2. Children are at higher risk than adults for obstruction of their airways. Which of the following are explanations for this? Select all that apply.
    1. Children do not chew their food as well.
    2. The diameter of the trachea is smaller.
    3. The trachea is shorter.
    4. The trachea is longer.

3. Which of the following assessment findings is an example of a child's body trying to naturally compensate during an acute respiratory illness?
    1. Slower respiratory rate
    2. Intercostal retractions
    3. Pale skin
    4. Coughing

4. A 2-year-old child hospitalized with pneumonia is assessed by the nurse. Which finding would cause the nurse to notify the physician?
   1. Respiratory rate of 24.
   2. Pulse oximeter reading of 92%.
   3. Retraction of the neck muscles when breathing.
   4. Lack of interest in food.

5. A parent states: "I know he is doing better because I can hear him breathing now." The nurse hears stridor when the child is taking a breath. The nurse's best response to the mother would be:
   1. "Maybe you can get some rest now."
   2. "That sound you hear means your child is having difficulty breathing."
   3. "I will let the physician know that he is doing better."
   4. "It means that the antibiotics are causing the secretions to become thinner."

6. A newborn is being assessed at 2 hours of age. Which of the following findings would alert the nurse to possible respiratory difficulty?
   1. Circumoral cyanosis
   2. Cyanosis of the hands and feet
   3. Pulse oximeter reading of 91%
   4. Upper airway secretions present

7. A parent calls the emergency department asking advice about her child's nosebleed. The child's nose has been bleeding for about 10 minutes. What direction would the nurse give the parent?
   1. Call back if it has not stopped in the next 5–10 minutes.
   2. Bring the child in for medical attention.
   3. Have the child lay down quietly until the bleeding stops.
   4. Have the child blow their nose to get any clots out and then apply pressure.

8. A 6-month-old is diagnosed with nasopharyngitis. Which of the following interventions would the nurse teach the family about caring for this child's illness? Select all that apply.
   1. Place a humidifier in the child's room.
   2. Administer aspirin if the child has a fever.
   3. Use saline nose drops prior to feedings.
   4. Administer an over-the-counter decongestant.

9. A child is being discharged after having a tonsillectomy. Which of the following nursing diagnoses will still apply after discharge?
   1. Ineffective Breathing Patterns Related to Airway Congestion
   2. Risk for Bleeding Related to Surgical Incision
   3. Knowledge Deficit Related to New Procedure
   4. Infection Related to Tonsillitis

10. When assessing a child postoperatively after having a tonsillectomy, the nurse notes that the child swallows frequently, but does not talk. The nurse understands that this most likely indicates:
    1. The child is in pain.
    2. The child has bleeding in the throat.
    3. The child is shy.
    4. The child is scared.

11. A child is diagnosed with epiglottitis. As the nurse enters the hospital room to perform the assessment, the nurse notices that the child is in the tripod position and drooling. The nurse should:
    1. Have the parent assist the child to lie down for the assessment.
    2. Pick the child up.
    3. Leave the child alone until the child falls asleep.
    4. Notify the physician.

12. The nurse teaches the parents of a 4-year-old child with a suspected diagnosis of epiglottitis why their child is not being fully assessed until the physician arrives. Which of the following would be reasons for this? Select all that apply.
    1. Crying would stimulate the airway.
    2. Oxygen consumption may increase with crying.
    3. Laryngospasm might occur.
    4. Airway occlusion is possible.

13. A child is suspected of swallowing a coin and is coughing and having color change. The trained health care provider knows that if the coin cannot be seen, the plan of care should be:
    1. Wait until the child loses consciousness, then initiate CPR.
    2. Call 911 immediately.
    3. Initiate the Heimlich maneuver.
    4. Use the finger sweep method.

14. A child is diagnosed at 6 years of age with cystic fibrosis. Which of the following might have been present earlier in the child's life to indicate the diagnosis?
    1. Being born 6 weeks premature.
    2. Having respiratory difficulty at birth.
    3. Presence of meconium ileus at birth.
    4. Presence of congenital hip dysplasia at birth.

15. The child with cystic fibrosis has many health problems that need to be addressed. Related to nutrition, which of the following would be recommended in this child's diet? Select all that apply.
    1. Low carbohydrate diet.
    2. Addition of pancreatic enzymes.
    3. High protein diet.
    4. Addition of vitamins.

CRITICAL THINKING EXERCISE

Read the case study. Answer the questions, keeping in mind the steps of the nursing process: assessing, diagnosing, planning, implementing, and evaluating.

A 2-month-old male infant is brought to the emergency department after being found without a pulse or respiratory effort by his 22-year-old parents. The family is of Native American descent. The doctors suspect the infant died of SIDS (sudden infant death syndrome). The parents are extremely distraught and express significant guilt over the death of their son. Tearfully, they ask the nurse, "What in the world happened to cause this?" They go on to say that even though he was born prematurely and was very small at birth, he had been doing well, eating and sleeping without difficulty. The mother reports: "We put him on his stomach in his bed as my mother-in-law told us to do. Did we do something wrong?"

1. Define SIDS.
2. Discuss the prevalence of SIDS.
3. From the preceding scenario, identify risk factors that may have predisposed the infant to SIDS.
4. Discuss the nurse's role in supporting this family.
5. Identify measures that parents should take to prevent the occurrence of SIDS.

Chapter 19

Care of the Child with Cardiovascular Disorders

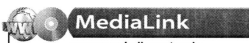

www.prenhall.com/towle

Use the address above to access the free, interactive Companion Website created for this textbook. Get hints, instant feedback to chapter-related NCLEX®-style questions. Link to other interesting sites.

Audio Glossary:

Use the Companion Website, or the CD-ROM disk enclosed with your textbook, to hear the pronunciation of key terms in the chapter.

Caring for a child with a cardiovascular disorder requires detailed assessments skills. Being able to detect a subtle change can mean avoidance of an emergency situation. Because of the chronic nature of many childhood cardiovascular disorders, the nurse must be knowledgeable enough about the common cardiovascular disorders during childhood to provide teaching to a child and their caregivers.

MATCHING

Match the term in the left column with the correct definition in the right column.

1. _____ Hyperlipidemia	A.	Involuntary movement
2. _____ Clubbing	B.	Wall between atrial chambers
3. _____ Coarctation	C.	Rheumatic rash
4. _____ Cardiomegaly	D.	Obstruction by suturing
5. _____ Septum	E.	Inflamed heart
6. _____ Chorea	F.	Aortic narrowing
7. _____ Pulmonary stenosis	G.	Elevated cholesterol
8. _____ Erythema marginatum	H.	Enlarged fingers due to hypoxia
9. _____ Ligation	I.	Enlarged heart
10. _____ Carditis	J.	Valve narrowing

FILL IN THE BLANKS

Fill in the blanks with the appropriate word or phrase.

1. Acute rheumatic fever is an inflammatory disorder that follows a group A beta-hemolytic _____ infection.

2. Nursing care for children with cardiac disorders includes assessing _____ status and _____ and _____ balance.

3. Polyarthritis of acute rheumatic fever responds best to the anti-inflammatory effects of _____.

4. Cyanosis around the mouth is known as _____ cyanosis.

5. The _____ _____ rate is used to assist in the diagnosis of _____ disease.

6. Children with _____ should be encouraged to consume a diet low in _____ and _____.

7. Antihypertensive medications are given to children with _____ hypertension.

8. The aorta and pulmonary artery are reversed in the disorder of

    _____ _____ _____ _____ _____.

9. With a coarctation of the aorta, the most common site of _____ is the aortic _____.

10. Most children with a ventricular septal defect have _____ symptoms.

MULTIPLE CHOICE

Circle the answer that best completes the following statements.

1. An infant is born with a congenital cardiac defect. The parents ask the nurse what might have caused this to happen. The nurse understands that there are several risk factors contributing to heart disorders. Select all the risk factors that apply to cardiovascular congenital defects.
    1. Advanced maternal age.
    2. Sibling with history of congenital heart defect.
    3. Advanced paternal age.
    4. Fetal exposure to rubella.

2. An infant is diagnosed with tetralogy of fallot (TOF). The nurse is preparing to discuss the defects that are encompassed in this diagnosis. Select all that apply.
    1. Right ventricular hypertrophy.
    2. Overriding aorta.
    3. Pulmonary stenosis.
    4. Ventricular septal defect.

3. The nurse is assessing a newborn infant. When palpating the pulses, the nurse notes that the femoral pulses are very weak. Based on this finding, what action should the nurse take first?
   1. Reassess within 1 hour to allow a transition period.
   2. Notify the physician.
   3. Assess the blood pressure in all four extremities.
   4. Count an apical pulse.

4. A key assessment finding difference in the child with pulmonary congestive heart failure compared to cardiac heart failure would include:
   1. Change in vital signs.
   2. Change in energy level.
   3. Presence of moist lung sounds.
   4. Age of child for diagnosis.

5. A child diagnosed with Kawasaki disease is exhibiting the following signs and symptoms: joint pain, fissures in skin, lips, hands and feet skin sloughing. What phase would the nurse anticipate this child is in?
   1. Acute
   2. Subacute
   3. Convalescent
   4. Chronic

6. Based on the treatment of Kawasaki disease with aspirin therapy, the nurse will teach the parents about which possible effect to watch for?
   1. Subnormal temperature
   2. Red rash
   3. Swollen joints
   4. Bleeding

7. When diagnosed with acute rheumatic fever, the parents of an 8-year-old female ask the nurse how their child could have acquired this disorder. The nurse's best response would be:
   1. "It is very contagious."
   2. "It may have occurred after a strep infection."
   3. "It is a viral illness, so it could have come from school."
   4. "Many children this age get this if they are active in sports."

8. Discharge teaching is being provided to the parents of a child recovering from acute rheumatic fever. The long-term teaching point that the nurse will discuss would be:
   1. No contact sports for 1 year.
   2. No immunizations for the next 6 months.
   3. Prophylactic antibiotics are needed before dental work.
   4. Long-term aspirin therapy will be prescribed.

9. The nurse advises the parents of a 2-week-old infant with a congenital cardiac defect resulting in congestive heart failure that they will need to have their child weighed each week. The primary rationale for this measure in this situation would be:
   1. The child will then be seen by a health care provider.
   2. To detect subtle fluid and electrolyte changes.
   3. To monitor the child's nutritional status.
   4. To assess medical treatment compliance.

10. When preparing to assess a blood pressure on an 11-month-old infant, the nurse must consider:
    1. The position of the infant.
    2. The time of day.
    3. The location of the strongest pulse.
    4. The size of the blood pressure cuff.

11. Select all of the following items that are included in the circulatory system.
    1. Heart
    2. Lungs
    3. Blood vessels
    4. Liver

12. In an infant with congenital heart disease, fluid retention may be evidenced by:
    1. Circumoral cyanosis.
    2. Orthopnea.
    3. Bulging fontanels.
    4. Lethargy.

13. In an infant with a congenital heart defect, restlessness, crying, and lethargy can be signs of:
    1. Pulmonary stenosis.
    2. Congestive heart failure.
    3. Ductus arteriosus.
    4. Hypoglycemia.

14. Which of the following disorders is the most common cause of acquired heart disease in children?
    1. Gastroenteritis
    2. Meningitis
    3. Epilepsy
    4. Conjunctival hyperemia

15. Which of the following would an infant be predisposed to experiencing based on the premise that the heart muscle fibers are not fully developed at birth?
    1. Kawasaki disease
    2. Rheumatic fever
    3. Ductus arteriosis
    4. Fluid and volume overload

CRITICAL THINKING EXERCISE

Read the case study. Answer the questions, keeping in mind the steps of the nursing process: assessing, diagnosing, planning, implementing, and evaluating.

An 18-month-old child is admitted to the hospital in congestive heart failure (CHF). The child was born with a ventricular septal defect. A surgical repair has not been performed. The child has a murmur and moist lung sounds and is pale and lethargic. The parents are very worried and confused about what is happening with their child.

1. Define CHF in a child.
2. Describe the target of treatment.
3. Identify three common nursing diagnoses for children with CHF.
4. Identify five nursing interventions for a child with CHF and provide rationale for each intervention.

Chapter 20

Care of the Child with Hematologic or Lymphatic Disorders

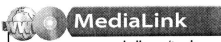

www.prenhall.com/towle

Use the address above to access the free, interactive Companion Website created for this textbook. Get hints, instant feedback to chapter-related NCLEX®-style questions. Link to other interesting sites.

Audio Glossary:

Use the Companion Website, or the CD-ROM disk enclosed with your textbook, to hear the pronunciation of key terms in the chapter.

Hematological and lymphatic disorders in children can be life-threatening. These disorders may be inherited or just occur. Because blood and lymph systems affect the entire body and its organs, these disorders can cause debilitating fatigue and death. Clients with hematologic and lymphatic disorders and their families require emotional support. The client and family require teaching as well as physical care and support of the client.

This study guide chapter will allow the reader to understand hematological and lymphatic disorders that affect the pediatric client. Knowledge of hematological and lymphatic disorders and how they are medically managed will allow the student to apply the nursing process in managing the pediatric client with these disorders.

MATCHING

Match the term in the left column with the correct definition in the right column.

1. _____ Hemophilia		A.	A process of naming the extent of the spread of cancer
2. _____ Sickle cell anemia		B.	A process by which RBCs are destroyed
3. _____ Erythropoiesis		C.	An X-linked recessive disorder
4. _____ Hemolysis		D.	A process by which RBCs are produced
5. _____ Purpura		E.	Disorder affecting the formation of hemoglobin
6. _____ Hemosiderosis		F.	Rash, blood cells leak into the skin
7. _____ Acute lymphoblastic anemia		G.	Iron overload
8. _____ Leukemia		H.	Disorder of abnormal hemoglobin synthesis
9. _____ Staging		I.	Cancer in which WBCs are abnormally increased
10. _____ Thalassemia		J.	Cancer cells develop in the bone marrow

FILL IN THE BLANKS

Fill in the blanks with the appropriate word or phrase.

1. The use of a(n) _____ in administering liquid iron will diminish the chances of staining the client's teeth.

2. Children with sickle cell anemia experience _____, and nurses must be attentive in managing it.

3. This nursing action, _____, is a priority for all clients, especially those with a diagnosis of leukemia.

4. A child with leukemia should avoid those individuals who are _____.

5. Vitamin C can increase the absorption of _____.

6. _____ are known as platelets.

MULTIPLE CHOICE

Circle the answer that best completes the following statements.

1. The mother of a 7-year-old client has brought her son in for routine blood work. The client has hemophilia. The mother mentions to the nurse that her son has enrolled in football. What teaching should the nurse provide?
   1. The nurse should teach the mother of the importance of monitoring her son for bruising.
   2. The nurse should inform the mother that her son should not engage in contact sports, which may cause bleeding.
   3. The nurse should inform the mother that exercise is important for her son.
   4. The nurse should inform the mother of frequent injuries that children sustain when playing football.

2. You are caring for an 11-year-old male client who has a medical diagnosis hemophilia. Upon your admission assessment, the client informs his mother he has had dark stools lately. You ask the client to describe his stools. The client replies, "They're very dark. They are black." What action should you take?
   1. Call the physician.
   2. Place a puritan hat in the toilet to obtain a stool specimen.
   3. Assess for rectal bleeding.
   4. Obtain a set of vital signs.

3. You are caring for a 5-year-old female client with a history of sickle cell anemia who was admitted for dehydration. You walk into the client's room and notice pallor and mild cyanosis. What action should you take?
   1. Increase IV fluids.
   2. Stop all IV fluids.
   3. Place the client on oxygen.
   4. Place the client in Trendelenburg position.

4. A pediatric client has been admitted with a medical diagnosis of hemosiderosis. The physician has ordered 1,000 mg of chewable Vitamin C to be given tid. The mother asks the nurse why her child is receiving Vitamin C. An appropriate response by the nurse would be:

   1. "The Vitamin C is prescribed to decrease your child's bleeding time."
   2. "The Vitamin C is given because the physician has noted a deficiency."
   3. "The Vitamin C is typically given to clients with hematomas."
   4. "The Vitamin C is given to help the body remove the excess iron."

5. On a routine pediatric examination of a client with a history of sickle cell anemia, the physician orders a pneumococcal vaccination. The mother questions the nurse as to why her son must have this vaccination. What would be an appropriate response by the nurse?

   1. "All pediatric clients should receive a pneumococcal vaccination."
   2. "With your son's history of sickle cell anemia, it is recommended he receive this vaccination to prevent infection, which could cause him to go into sickle cell crisis."
   3. "The sickle cell anemia predisposes your son to infection. This vaccination will protect him from obtaining pneumonia."
   4. "The pneumococcal vaccination should be administered annually to all pediatric clients with a history of hematological disorders."

6. A 5-year-old female client is admitted with shortness of breath and nonproductive cough, which has increased in severity over the past few days. The client has a history of thalassemia. What physician's orders would you expect?

   1. Oxygen, IV access, I & O, and chest x-ray stat.
   2. Oxygen and stat IV Lasix.
   3. IV access, I & O, and serum electrolytes.
   4. IV access and oxygen.

7. You are working in the emergency department when a 10-year-old male client is admitted for a laceration to the right forearm. The client states he was playing with his friends and fell on a tree limb. The mother informs you her son has a history of hemophilia. What action should you take?

   1. Obtain a heart rate, temperature, and apply sterile gauze to the laceration.
   2. Apply an ice pack to the laceration and obtain a set of vital signs.
   3. Apply sterile gauze and pressure to the laceration, elevate the extremity, and call for assistance.
   4. Apply sterile gauze to the site, call for assistance, and offer emotional support.

8. A mother with a 2-year-old daughter who is diagnosed with iron deficiency anemia does not understand why her daughter's hemoglobin levels are low. The nurse questions the mother about the child's diet within the past 24 hours. Which of the following food choices indicates a need for further education?

   1. Milk, fruit-loops cereal, hot dog, grapes, green beans, apple juice, macaroni and cheese, and peas
   2. Milk, cheeseburger, orange slices, apple juice, toast with grape jelly, chicken, broccoli, and mashed potatoes
   3. Oatmeal, orange juice, raisins, macaroni with cheese, chicken, broccoli, milk, and peanut butter and jelly sandwich
   4. Scrambled eggs, toast, milk, peanut butter and jelly sandwich, apple juice, hamburger, spinach, and mashed potatoes

9. You are caring for a school-age client with a history of ITP. The client is scheduled to have a tonsillectomy and is receiving a preop infusion of platelets. The client states, "My arms itch." What action should you take?
   1. Assess the infusion site.
   2. Stop the infusion immediately.
   3. Increase the IV infusion rate.
   4. Call the physician.

10. In planning your care for a 10-year-old client with ALL who is receiving chemotherapy, which nursing diagnosis would be appropriate for this client?
    1. Development: Delayed Risk for Related to Medical Treatment
    2. Anxiety Related to Medical Ttreatment
    3. Health Maintenance, Ineffective Related to Disease Process
    4. Infection, Risk for Related to Medical Treatment

11. A 17-year-old client who is being treated for Hodgkin's lymphoma is experiencing alopecia. The client is withdrawn and not interested in talking to his friends on the telephone. Which would be an appropriate nursing diagnosis for this client?
    1. Health Maintenance, Ineffective Related to Medical Treatment
    2. Body Image, Disturbed Related to Alopecia
    3. Diversional Activity, Deficient Related to Nontherapeutic Communication
    4. Grieving, Dysfunctional Related to Limited Contact with Peers

12. The mother of a teenage client is questioning the nurse regarding the staging for her son's Hodgkin's lymphoma diagnosis. She states, "What is the difference between stage II and stage III?" An appropriate response by the nurse would be:
    1. "Stage II indicates the disease is in two lymph nodes, and Stage III indicates three."
    2. "Stage II indicates the disease is in the neck region, and Stage III indicates it is in the thoracic area."
    3. "Stage II indicates the disease is in the lymph nodes on one side of the diaphragm, and Stage III indicates it is on both sides of the diaphragm."
    4. "Stage II indicates the location of the disease is in a specific organ, and Stage III indicates it has spread from the organ to the surrounding tissue."

13. The father of a client with sickle cell disease does not understand why his son is experiencing pain in his joints. An appropriate response by the nurse would be:
    1. "Your son is experiencing pain because his joints are infected."
    2. "Your son must have fallen at home, which is causing him pain."
    3. "Your son's joints are painful because the sickle cells accumulate at the joint and cause swelling."
    4. "Your son's joints are arthritic, which is a complication of sickle cell anemia."

14. A mother who has a child with terminal Hodgkin's lymphoma is concerned about her child's decreased appetite. She states, "I prepare a meal, and she takes a few bites and complains of being tired and will not eat anymore." Which of the following comments by the nurse would be appropriate?
    1. "Your daughter's disease has progressed to where she will not eat much."
    2. "Eating causes fatigue. Prepare frequent nutritious meals and snacks."
    3. "Prepare large meals early in the day. She will eat when she smells the aroma of food."
    4. "Prepare various types of meals with a variety of foods and encourage her to get up and eat with the family."

15. The mother of a 2-year-old child with iron deficiency anemia is complaining of her daughter's frequent bouts of constipation. Which of the following statements would offer the most beneficial information for the mother so she may manage this situation?
    1. "Iron supplements cause constipation; there is little that can be done about it."
    2. "Iron supplements cause constipation and gastritis. You should call your physician."
    3. "Constipation is an abnormal complication of iron deficiency anemia. You should contact your physician."
    4. "Iron supplements may cause constipation. Increase your daughter's fluid intake, offer high fiber foods, and make sure she receives daily exercise."

16. A 10-year-old male client is hospitalized while receiving chemotherapy for acute myelogenous leukemia (AML). The mother has brought in fast food and drink. You are caring for this client and enter the room to perform your assessment. You notice the client has eaten and drunk what was brought in by his mother. You ask the client how much he ate and drank. The mother questions why this is important. An appropriate response would be:
    1. "I have to monitor what is eaten by my clients."
    2. "I record how much your son has eaten and drunk. One reason is to monitor his kidney function."
    3. "Every client has their intake, output, and amount of food eaten monitored."
    4. "I want to make sure your son is eating a balanced diet."

CRITICAL THINKING EXERCISE

Read the case study. Answer the questions, keeping in mind the steps of the nursing process: assessing, diagnosing, planning, implementing, and evaluating.

A 10-month-old-infant has just been diagnosed with sickle cell crisis and is resting quietly after receiving IV medication. The mother is crying and states, "I'll never be able to take care of him at home. What if he has this pain again?"

1. What education should be provided to the mother so she may prevent an episode of sickle cell crisis?

2. When the mother returns home with her son, what signs and symptoms should she report to her pediatrician?

3. What measures can the mother implement to manage her son's pain while at home?

4. What is vaso-occlusive sickle cell crisis?

Chapter 21

Care of the Child with Immune Disorders

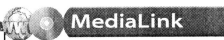

www.prenhall.com/towle

Use the address above to access the free, interactive Companion Website created for this textbook. Get hints, instant feedback to chapter-related NCLEX®-style questions. Link to other interesting sites.

Audio Glossary:

Use the Companion Website, or the CD-ROM disk enclosed with your textbook, to hear the pronunciation of key terms in the chapter.

The immune system provides protection against infection and disease. A functioning immune system is vital for one to exist. If the immune system does not function properly, it can lead to diseases and disorders.

This study guide chapter allows the reader to understand a variety of disorders related to the immune system that affect the pediatric client. Knowledge of immune disorders and how they are medically managed will allow the student to apply the nursing process in managing the pediatric client with these disorders.

MATCHING

Match the term in the left column with the correct definition in the right column.

1. _____ Natural immunity	A.	Process that causes rejection of transplanted organs	
2. _____ Acquired immunity	B.	Immunizations provide this type of immunity	
3. _____ Cell-mediated immunity	C.	Small doses can accomplish this	
4. _____ Active immunity	D.	Also known as "thrush"	
5. _____ HIV	E.	Autoimmune disorder affecting connective tissue	
6. _____ Candidiasis	F.	Autoimmune disorder affecting joints	
7. _____ Juvenile rheumatoid arthritis	G.	Acquired by exposure over time	
8. _____ Hepatomegaly	H.	Enlarged liver	
9. _____ Lupus	I.	Is a retrovirus	
10. _____ Desensitization	J.	Present at birth	

FILL IN THE BLANKS

Fill in the blanks with the appropriate word or phrase.

1. The primary role of the immune system is to eliminate _____ substances.

2. _____, a type of fungal infection, can be found in the diaper region.

3. This type of test, _____ Advance Rapid HIV-1/2 Antibody Test, can produce results in 20 minutes.

4. _____ and _____ cause inflammation, which may cause pain.

5. Obtaining a thorough _____ is important to determine a client's allergies.

6. A newborn is protected by _____ _____.

MULTIPLE CHOICE

Circle the answer that best completes the following statements.

1. A mother who is visiting the pediatrician with her son states to the nurse, "I don't understand why my doctor wants me to have an HIV test." You know this mother is expecting her second child in approximately 4 months. Which response would be appropriate?
    1. "HIV can be transmitted to the baby, and your physician would like you to be tested."
    2. "HIV is very prevalent today, and the physician must report all known cases to the health department."
    3. "The physician would like to know if he must implement standard precautions when he delivers your baby."
    4. "HIV is easily transmitted, and all people who visit their physician are required to be tested."

2. The mother of an 18-month-old male client is concerned because he has just been diagnosed with HIV. When teaching the mother concerning management of her son's disease, which of the following is important to include?
    1. Bonding with both parents.
    2. Ensuring proper oral hygiene on a daily basis.
    3. Frequent hand washing.
    4. Monitoring intake and output.

3. The mother of a 2-year-old male client with a diagnosis of HIV is visiting the pediatrician. While conversing with the mother, the nurse learns the client's vocabulary consists of two words, "mama" and "dada." Which of the following statements is correct regarding this client?
   1. Two-year-old children typically have one to two words, which consist of their entire vocabulary.
   2. Children with a diagnosis of HIV/AIDs may have developmental delays.
   3. Toddlers can be reluctant to speak because they are temperamental.
   4. This client should be referred to a speech therapist.

4. A 4-year-old client has been brought into the pediatrician's office for a complaint of leg pain. The father informs the nurse the client has been limping when ambulating and complaining of pain in the right lower extremity. The father and client deny any injury to the extremity. The nurse suspects which of the following?
   1. Growth pains.
   2. Problems with the client's growth plate.
   3. Injury to the right lower extremity.
   4. Possible juvenile rheumatoid arthritis.

5. A 5-year-old male client has a medical diagnosis of JRA. The mother is concerned about her son's pain. She asks the nurse about alternative methods she can utilize at home. Which of the following would be appropriate?
   1. Ice packs to joints and increased fluids.
   2. Warm baths and ROM exercises.
   3. Warm baths and frequent walks.
   4. Ice packs to joints and moderate weight lifting exercises.

6. A mother of a 15-year-old male client calls the physician's office and asks to speak with the nurse. The mother informs the nurse her son, who has a history of lupus, has gained weight over recent weeks, has increased acne, and has been very irritable. The nurse suspects this client is on which of the following medications?
   1. NSAIDS
   2. Salicylates
   3. Beta-blockers
   4. Corticosteroids

7. You are caring for a 16-year-old male client who has a medical diagnosis of lupus. He is doing well and will possibly go home in a few days. The client has been complaining about weight gain and increased acne, which is due to his current medication regimen. Which nursing diagnosis is appropriate for this client?
   1. Nutrition Imbalance; Less than Body Requirements
   2. Coping, Defensive Related to Acne
   3. Body Image, Disturbed Related to Weight Gain and Acne
   4. Energy Field Disturbance, Related to Weight Gain

8. A young male client is brain dead, and the nurse approaches the parents about organ donation. The parents are divorced and have remarried. The nurse understands that she must obtain consent for the organ donation from which of the following?
    1. The parent the child lives with.
    2. Both parents.
    3. The parent who is present when the nurse is obtaining the consent.
    4. One parent; it does not matter which parent.

9. The nurse is informing the parents of a 2-year-old child of the postoperative management of their son after a kidney transplant. The father asks the nurse what types of medications he will be receiving. Which of the following would be an appropriate response?
    1. Antihypertensives
    2. Tricyclic antidepressants
    3. Immunosuppressives
    4. NSAIDS

10. The nurse is preparing discharge instructions for a 2-year-old client who received a kidney transplant. Which of the following are important to include in the client's/parental education?
    1. The client should avoid individuals who are ill.
    2. The client should have frequent monitoring of heart rate every 8 hours.
    3. The client should play often with peers.
    4. The client should remain on anticoagulants.

11. A 6-year-old female client who is allergic to latex has just received her dinner tray. The nurse is assisting the client with her tray and notices there is a food on the client's tray that should be avoided. Which should this client avoid?
    1. Apples
    2. Bananas
    3. Pretzels
    4. Milk

12. Which nursing diagnosis would be appropriate for a client with a diagnosis of JRA?
    1. Nutrition Imbalance: More than Body Requirements
    2. Nutrition Imbalance: Less than Body Requirements
    3. Aspiration: Risk for Related to Disease Process
    4. Activity Intolerance: Risk for Related to Disease Process

13. When educating the parents of a 10-year-old female client with a diagnosis of JRA who is to remain on strict bed rest for a week, it is important to include:
    1. Frequent exercise.
    2. Cold packs to joints every 8 hours.
    3. Turning and ROM.
    4. Increased fluids.

14. A female client who has tested positive for HIV does not understand why she must have a cesarean section. Which response by the nurse would be appropriate?
   1. "Your baby may contact the HIV virus when she is delivered through the birth canal."
   2. "Your baby will have the HIV virus and must be delivered quickly so the physician may assess the neonate."
   3. "Your baby must be delivered early, and this is the best method."
   4. "The physician prefers this method for clients who have a history of HIV."

15. You are caring for a 13-year-old client with a diagnosis of lupus. The physician orders a fasting glucose before each meal. The mother questions the nurse as to why this must be done. The best response would be:
   1. "Diabetes typically appears at this age, so we are going to monitor your daughter while she is here."
   2. "Your daughter's glucose must have been high, and the physician would like to monitor it."
   3. "Your daughter's pancreas must not be functioning correctly."
   4. "Your daughter is receiving corticosteroids, which may raise her glucose levels."

16. A mother brings her 14-year-old daughter into the pediatrician's office because her daughter has been complaining of numbness, pain, and pallor of her hands for the past few weeks. The mother states, "She refuses to wear her mittens when she goes to school." The nurse suspects:
   1. Carpal tunnel syndrome.
   2. Raynaud's phenomenon.
   3. Phantom pain.
   4. Radial palsy.

CRITICAL THINKING EXERCISE

Read the case study. Answer the questions, keeping in mind the steps of the nursing process: assessing, diagnosing, planning, implementing, and evaluating.

You are caring for a female client who is pregnant. She has recently been diagnosed with HIV. This is her first pregnancy. What education is important for this client?

1. What type of delivery should this client expect?
2. How should this client feed her neonate?
3. How may she prevent transmission in the future?
4. What can be done to prevent the transmission of the HIV virus to the fetus?

Chapter 22

Care of the Child with Gastrointestinal Disorders

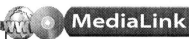

MediaLink

www.prenhall.com/towle

Use the address above to access the free, interactive Companion Website created for this textbook. Get hints, instant feedback to chapter-related NCLEX®-style questions. Link to other interesting sites.

Audio Glossary:

Use the Companion Website, or the CD-ROM disk enclosed with your textbook, to hear the pronunciation of key terms in the chapter.

The gastrointestinal system provides energy to the body by digesting food while eliminating wastes. Clients' gastrointestinal disorders may occur because of congenital abnormalities, problems with absorption, or motility.

This study guide chapter will allow the reader to understand gastrointestinal disorders that affect the pediatric client. Knowledge of gastrointestinal disorders and how they are medically managed will allow the student to apply the nursing process in managing the pediatric client with these disorders.

MATCHING

Match the term in the left column with the correct definition in the right column.

1. _____ Kwashiorkor	A.	Inflammation of the liver
2. _____ Lactose intolerance	B.	Random inflammation of the GI tract
3. _____ Scurvy	C.	Inflammation of the stomach
4. _____ Hepatitis	D.	Inability to digest gluten
5. _____ Cleft palate	E.	Inflammation and sloughing of the large intestinal mucosa
6. _____ Esophageal atresia	F.	Protein deficiency
7. _____ Gastroenteritis	G.	Inability to digest lactose
8. _____ Crohn's disease	H.	A blind pouch at the end of the esophagus
9. _____ Ulcerative colitis	I.	A lack of Vitamin C in the diet
10. _____ Celiac disease	J.	An opening at the roof of the mouth

FILL IN THE BLANKS

Fill in the blanks with the appropriate word or phrase.

1. Parents of a newborn with a cleft lip and palate will need _____ and _____ in caring for their child.

2. A sudden release of RLQ pain for the client with appendicitis indicates _____ _____.

3. Fluid leak around a stoma can cause _____.

4. The child with _____ may become mentally dull.

5. The mnemonic SIRES stands for: S_____, I_____, R_____, E_____, and S_____.

6. A connection between the yolk sac and the intestine, which causes a pouch, is called a(n) _____ _____.

7. _____ _____ is more common in boys and commonly occurs with congenital heart defects, Down syndrome, and other neurological syndromes.

MULTIPLE CHOICE

Circle the answer that best completes the following statements.

1. You are caring for a newborn client with a diagnosis of cleft lip and palate. The mother is feeding the newborn and complains the newborn chokes frequently when feeding him. What education does the mother require?
   1. How to feed the newborn with a straw.
   2. How to feed the newborn with a Breck feeder.
   3. How to provide TPN via a central venous catheter.
   4. How to encourage sucking so the oral muscles are strong prior to surgery.

2. You are caring for a 2-year-old client with a diagnosis of gastroenteritis. The mother asks you what she might expect regarding the medical treatment for her son. Which response is appropriate?
   1. IV fluids, blood cultures, and chest x-ray
   2. Chest x-ray, upper GI, and electrolytes
   3. Serum electrolytes, IV fluids, and I & O
   4. I & O, IV fluids, and stool for occult blood

3. You are caring for a 13-year-old male client who was admitted to the pediatric unit complaining of abdominal pain. Upon your admission assessment, you learn the client had a sudden onset of abdominal pain and nausea, which progressed to vomiting and a temperature of 100.2°F. The client requests a drink of water. Which action should you take?
   1. Inform the client you have not received the physician's orders, and at this moment, he must remain NPO.
   2. Give the client ice chips.
   3. Give the client a glass of water.
   4. Inform the client he may only have clear liquids at this time.

4. The physician assesses a 13-year-old male client who was admitted to the pediatric unit complaining of abdominal pain and states, "He has rebound tenderness. I'll write an order for a consent." The mother asks, "What is rebound tenderness?" The best response by the nurse would be:
   1. "Rebound tenderness is any tenderness in the abdomen."
   2. "It's just a medical term physicians use to describe the adipose tissue in the abdomen."
   3. "It means there is pain on release of pressure to the area."
   4. "It means there is inflammation at the area."

5. A 16-year-old female client has a recent diagnosis of Crohn's disease. The mother is concerned because her daughter will not go out on dates due to a possible episode of diarrhea. Which nursing diagnosis would be appropriate for this client?
   1. Nutrition: Malabsorption Related to Diagnosis of Crohn's Disease
   2. Self-Care Deficit Related to Toileting
   3. Coping, Ineffective Related to Complications of Disease Process
   4. Maladjustment, Related to Crohn's Disease

6. You are caring for a 5-year-old female client who was admitted for dehydration. She has a history of celiac disease. She is expected to go home tomorrow, and the physician has ordered a regular diet to assess if she's able to tolerate it. Her breakfast tray arrives with oatmeal, 2% milk, eggs, bacon, a plain bagel, and orange juice. Which food is contraindicated for the client with celiac disease?
   1. Orange juice
   2. Bagel
   3. Protein
   4. Oatmeal

7. In teaching the parents of a client with a recent diagnosis of celiac disease, the mother does not understand why her son will not be able to eat wheat for the rest of his life. Which of the following would be important to mention to the parents?
   1. "Your son will never be able to digest wheat."
   2. "Avoidance of foods that contain gluten is important because a person could develop gastrointestinal cancer."
   3. "Avoidance of these foods is important or your son will have embarrassing bouts of diarrhea."
   4. "Your son needs to avoid these foods because the physician prescribed this diet regimen."

8. The discharge instruction for a Hispanic client with a medical diagnosis of rickets instructs the client to be outdoors daily. The father, who speaks English well asks, "Why does my son need to go outside every day?" The best response by the nurse would be:
   1. "Because it's important your son has daily exercise."
   2. "Because the physician recommends it."
   3. "Because Vitamin C is better absorbed when your child is exercising."
   4. "Because Vitamin D is obtained from the sun."

9. You receive a 2-month-old male client with a diagnosis of "failure to thrive." When the parents arrive on the unit, which of the following would cause concern?
    1. The mother is crying and holding her infant while the father is sitting in a chair.
    2. The mother ignores the infant, and the father appears to be frustrated.
    3. The father asking, "What is wrong with my son?" while comforting the mother.
    4. The father and mother are concerned and cuddling their son.

10. You are caring for a 3-week-old male infant with a diagnosis of biliary atresia. During your shift while changing the infant's diapers, you notice his stools are clay colored and his urine is dark, tea colored. What should you do?
    1. Report your findings to the RN and the physician because this is a typical finding with biliary atresia.
    2. Report your findings immediately to the physician.
    3. Call a fellow nurse to assess the diapers.
    4. Call your supervisor.

11. You are caring for a 10-year-old male client who was admitted from the emergency department after experiencing a seizure. When obtaining a history, the mother states her son attended a birthday party and is suspected of ingesting a soda pop. This client has a history of PKU. What nursing interventions should you implement for this client?
    1. Diversional activities.
    2. Fluid restrictions.
    3. Complete bed rest.
    4. Seizure precautions.

12. You receive a 5-week-old male client from the emergency department with a diagnosis of dehydration. While performing your admission assessment, the mother informs you her son has had increasing episodes of vomiting. The mother states, "When he vomits it goes clear across the room." You suspect the client may have which of the following?
    1. Pyloric stenosis.
    2. GERD.
    3. Esophageal atresia.
    4. Colitis.

13. You receive a 3-year-old male client with a sudden onset of abdominal pain and vomiting. He has IV fluids infusing and ambulates to the bathroom with his mother. You inform the mother not to flush the stool. After the child has returned to bed, you notice red, gelatinous, stool in the toilet. Which action should you take?
    1. Call another nurse and ask her opinion.
    2. Call the RN and inform him/her of your findings.
    3. Send the stool to the lab.
    4. Flush the toilet, and obtain a weight on the client.

14. You are discharging a 2-year-old female client after she has recovered from a bout of gastroenteritis. The client has a 1-year-old and a 5-year-old sibling at home. The mother states she is happy her daughter will be home for Christmas. Knowing children of this age are at risk for poisonings, which of the following household items might you warn the mother about?
    1. Ornaments on the Christmas tree.
    2. Toilet paper.
    3. OTC medicines.
    4. Poinsettias.

15. You are working for the local health department and are assisting an RN in evaluating homes for lead. Which of the following areas or items in the house would you want to evaluate?
    1. Paint and water.
    2. Water heater and air conditioner.
    3. Furnace and air conditioner.
    4. Mattresses and carpet.

16. A mother brings her 4-week-old infant into the pediatrician's office because her skin color has changed, and the mother has noticed bruising on the infant's extremities and changes in her infant's stools. Upon questioning the mother, you learn the infant's stools are whitish-gray and are thick even though the mother is breastfeeding. Which laboratory tests would you anticipate the pediatrician to order?
    1. Liver enzymes and urinalysis.
    2. Bleeding time and stool culture.
    3. Liver enzymes and bleeding time.
    4. Bleeding time and upper GI series.

17. You are a nurse working in the pediatrician's office. A mother has brought in her 15-month-old son because she noticed a lump in his groin. While assessing the client, flat on the examination table, you notice nothing in the groin area. The mother states, "I noticed it a few nights ago when he stood to get out of the bathtub." Which action should you perform next?
    1. Palpate both groin areas.
    2. Listen for bowel sounds in all four quadrants.
    3. Auscultate the client's lungs.
    4. Assist the client to a standing position.

18. A father has brought his 4-year-old son into the pediatrician's office because of his son's complaint of abdominal pain. The father states, "He will sit on the toilet for a long time and sometimes have a large bowel movement and sometimes it's diarrhea." What other information would the nurse want to know?
    1. "How long has this been happening?"
    2. "What has he eaten in the past 48 to 72 hours?"
    3. "Is there a family history of colon cancer?"
    4. "What types of fluids does the client intake in a 24-hour period of time?"

Read the case study. Answer the questions, keeping in mind the steps of the nursing process: assessing, diagnosing, planning, implementing, and evaluating.

You are working in an inner-city clinic. A mother brings in her 3-year-old son, who has had diarrhea and abdominal pain for the past 2 days. When you assess the client, he appears lethargic and pale. The mother is of Hispanic descent and states they have just returned from visiting her parents in Mexico. The client's vital signs are T 100.2°F, P 86, R 24, B/P 84/44.

1. What should your next action be?
2. What other information would you want to obtain from the mother?
3. What type of labs do you anticipate the physician or nurse practitioner to order?
4. What action do you anticipate the nurse practitioner or the physician to implement next?

Chapter 23

Care of the Child with Genitourinary Disorders

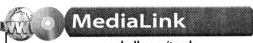

The urinary system functions to remove wastes from the body, maintain homeostasis, regulate blood pressure and calcium metabolism, and stimulate the production of erythrocytes. Because of the significant functions of the urinary system, disorders may cause significant health disorders and place the pediatric client at risk.

The reproductive organs when mature will assist the client in achieving childbirth. The male and female reproductive organs produce, protect, and transport ova or sperm; provide sexual pleasure; and regulate hormones within the body. Anomalies of the urinary system can also affect the reproductive system.

This study guide chapter will allow the reader to understand urinary and reproductive disorders that affect the pediatric client. Knowledge of urinary and reproductive disorders and how they are medically managed will allow the student to apply the nursing process in managing the pediatric client with these disorders.

MATCHING

Match the term in the left column with the correct definition in the right column.

1. _____ Hydrocele   A. Undescended testicle
2. _____ Testicular torsion B. Tumor of the kidney
3. _____ Wilms' tumor   C. Twisted testicle
4. _____ Cryptorchidism   D. Accumulation of fluid in the scrotum
5. _____ Peritoneal dialysis E. Inflammation of the kidney pelvis
6. _____ ARF   F. Sudden onset of reduced kidney function
7. _____ Ascites   G. Bladder infection
8. _____ Pyelonephritis   H. Edema in the abdomen
9. _____ Hematuria   I. Infuse dialysate into the peritoneal cavity
10. _____ Cystitis   J. Blood in the urine

5. A 6-year-old male client has a diagnosis of nephritic syndrome. The physician has ordered a 24-hour urine. The mother inquires as to why the client's urine must be obtained over a long period of time. Which would be an appropriate response?
   1. "A collection over 24 hours allows the physician to determine how inflamed your son's kidneys are and how best to treat it."
   2. "A collection over 24 hours allows the lab to have enough urine to test."
   3. "A 24-hour urine allows for the protein to settle in the container so it may be analyzed."
   4. "A 24-hour urine is a more accurate test than a urinalysis."

6. You are caring for a 4-year-old male client with a diagnosis of Wilms' tumor. You are going off your shift and saying good-bye to the client. The night shift nurse enters the room and auscultates the client's abdomen for bowel sounds. She then attempts to palpate the abdomen. What should you do?
   1. Nothing; allow her to complete her assessment.
   2. Interrupt her and inform her she should not palpate the abdomen.
   3. Instruct her on how to palpate this client's abdomen.
   4. Inform her that she is to palpate the abdomen first, then auscultate for bowel sounds.

7. You are caring for a postop client who has undergone a nephrectomy for a Wilms' tumor. What specifically should you assess regarding this client?
   1. I & O, serum glucose, and temperature
   2. I & O, hematuria, and temperature
   3. I & O, temperature, and BUN
   4. I & O, daily weight, and blood pressure

8. Which of the following contributes to enuresis?
   1. Inadequate fluid intake
   2. Stressors
   3. Poor nutrition
   4. Proteinuria

9. A 9-year-old client with end-stage renal failure requests a popsicle. You are determining whether the client may have this popsicle because:
   1. The client is on a fluid restriction.
   2. This is not allowed on a renal diet.
   3. The client is not allowed a high-caloric food item.
   4. The client is not on a clear liquid diet.

10. A 2-month-old male client is being seen by the pediatrician. The mother states, "The last time we were here the doctor was concerned about one of his testicles not being where it should be." The mother states, "He is supposed to have an oorchy hexy, whatever that is." Which of the following statements by the nurse would be appropriate?
    1. "An orchiopexy is the testicle is removed."
    2. "An orchiopexy is when the testicle is pulled down from the abdomen and placed in the scrotum."
    3. "A cryptorchidism is when the testicle is removed."
    4. "I am not familiar with oorchy hexy."

11. The physician has discussed placing an adolescent client on birth control pills to assist with metrorrhagia. The mother does not understand why her daughter is to be placed on birth control pills. The best response by the nurse would be:
    1. "Your daughter is at the age in which she may be sexually active."
    2. "Is your daughter sexually active?"
    3. "The birth control pills with help regulate her periods."
    4. "The oirth control pills will help with the painful periods."

12. The physician has ordered a pregnancy test on a 15-year-old client because of amenorrhea. The physician has ordered this test because she has:
    1. not had a period.
    2. nausea and vomiting.
    3. been sexually active.
    4. gained weight.

13. The mother of a 16-year-old client who has vaginitis due to trichomoniasis is questioning why the physician has ordered a pregnancy test. The most appropriate response by the nurse would be:
    1. "The physician is concerned about possible uterine infection."
    2. "Trichomoniasis is a sexually transmitted disease; the physician wants to see if your daughter may be pregnant as well."
    3. "Trichomoniasis can occur during the first trimester."
    4. "Vaginitis can increase your daughter's chances of becoming pregnant."

14. A 9-year-old female client has been admitted with a diagnosis of vaginitis. The nurse observes for signs and symptoms of:
    1. Sepsis
    2. Amenorrhea
    3. Sexual abuse
    4. Nephritis

15. A female client with a diagnosis of vaginitis is going home. What important information should the nurse include in her discharge instructions?
    1. Avoid sexual activity for 10 days.
    2. Wipe the perineum from front to back.
    3. Increase her fluid intake.
    4. Avoid constipation.

16. A 6-year-old male client is admitted with a diagnosis of UTI. The client is complaining of right flank pain. The pediatrician has ordered an IVP, which showed hydronephrosis. The mother asks, "What is hydronephrosis?" The best answer would be:
    1. "It's a condition in which the kidney has extra fluid."
    2. "It's a condition that means your son has a kidney infection."
    3. "Hydronephrosis is a condition that causes a backflow of urine."
    4. "Hydronephrosis is a urinary tract infection."

CRITICAL THINKING EXERCISE

Read the case study. Answer the questions, keeping in mind the steps of the nursing process: assessing, diagnosing, planning, implementing, and evaluating.

You have received an 8-year-old female client from the emergency department with a diagnosis of vaginitis. You have obtained a medical history, and her vital signs are T 100.2°F, P 84, R 16, and B/P 96/44. You are performing a physical examination and note bruising on the child's wrists and thighs.

1. What should you document regarding your findings?
2. What action should you take?
3. What education should you provide for this client?
4. How can you make this client comfortable?

Chapter 24

Care of the Child with Integumentary Disorders

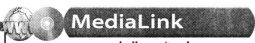
MediaLink
www.prenhall.com/towle

Use the address above to access the free, interactive Companion Website created for this textbook. Get hints, instant feedback to chapter-related NCLEX®-style questions. Link to other interesting sites.

Audio Glossary:
Use the Companion Website, or the CD-ROM disk enclosed with your textbook, to hear the pronunciation of key terms in the chapter.

Skin serves several functions. The main function of the skin is to protect the body from pathogens that may cause infections. Temperature regulation can also be influenced by the skin when the blood vessels dilate (allowing heat to dissipate from the body), and through perspiration (allowing evaporation of fluids). Production of sebum creates an oily barrier that helps prevent fluid loss. Sensory receptors provide information about pain, touch, pressure, and temperature. Sensory input is delivered to the brain so the body can adapt to the outside environment. The outer layer of the skin participates in the production of vitamin D.

This study guide chapter will allow the reader to understand integumentary disorders that affect the pediatric client. Knowledge of integumentary disorders and how they are medically managed will allow the student to apply the nursing process in managing the pediatric client with these disorders.

MATCHING

Match the term in the left column with the correct definition in the right column.

1. _____ Tinea pedis   A.   Herpes virus, "fever blister"

2. _____ Contact dermatitis   B.   Warts

3. _____ Eczema   C.   Skin fungi, "ringworm"

4. _____ Acne vulgaris   D.   Inflamed skin, due to irritant or allergen

5. _____ Pediculosis   E.   Skin condition, affects adolescents

6. _____ Dermatophytes   F.   Chronic, inflamed skin

7. _____ Scabies   G.   Lice

8. _____ Papillomavirus   H.   Skin infection caused by streptococci or staphylococci

9. _____ Herpes simplex I   I.   Athlete's foot

10. _____ Impetigo   J.   Skin is infected by a mite

8. A 4-year-old male is admitted to the pediatric unit with a diagnosis of asthma. Upon admission, the nurse notes scaly, whitish-pink areas on the forearms of this client. The nurse suspects:
   1. Contact dermatitis.
   2. Seborrheic dermatitis.
   3. Eczema.
   4. Impetigo.

9. You are caring for a 9-year-old client who has a history of eczema. A new LPN/LVN asks you, "What is eczema?" Your best response would be which of the following?
   1. "Eczema is caused by allergens."
   2. "Eczema is a condition caused by an autoimmune response to the environment."
   3. "It is a condition some clients obtain when admitted to the hospital."
   4. "It is caused by exposure to mites."

10. A mother states that her 9-year-old son always wears long sleeves, even in the summer. The son has a history of eczema to the upper extremities. A proper nursing diagnosis for this client would be:
    1. Skin Integrity, Impaired Related to Medical Condition.
    2. Body Image Disturbed, Related to Eczema.
    3. Knowledge Deficient, Related to Management of Eczema.
    4. Noncompliance, Related to Management of Eczema.

11. The mother of a 5-year-old female client with a diagnosis of eczema is frustrated because she states, "We are applying ointment and keeping her skin moist. Nothing seems to help." What information would help the nurse provide other suggestions to help manage this problem?
    1. The child's weight, food and fluid intake.
    2. The child's exposure to extreme temperatures.
    3. The home environment, such as pets, carpet, types of clothing, and use of detergents.
    4. The types of soaps and detergents used at home.

12. Which type of clothing should a client with a history of eczema wear?
    1. Wool and cotton clothing.
    2. Loose-fitting, soft clothing.
    3. Denim and wool clothing.
    4. Formfitting cotton clothing.

13. You are educating a 15-year-old female client on how to manage her acne. Which of the following would you include in your information?
    1. Use of oil-free cosmetics.
    2. Use of mild soaps.
    3. Use of mild abrasive cleansers.
    4. Use of alcohol topically to dry lesions.

14. A 16-year-old client and her mother are visiting the dermatologist for treatment of the client's acne. The dermatologist informs the client and her mother that she is going to prescribe Accutane to treat the acne. The physician orders a pregnancy test. The mother is very upset and asks the nurse why this test is ordered. The best response would be:
    1. "Is your daughter sexually active?"
    2. "Your daughter must be sexually active."
    3. "This medication is contraindicated if the client is pregnant."
    4. "I do not know why the physician has ordered this test."

15. An adolescent client is visiting the physician for treatment of his acne. The nursing diagnosis that would be most appropriate for this client is:
    1. Confusion, Acute Related to Treatment Regime.
    2. Health Maintenance Ineffective, Related to Proper Hygiene.
    3. Noncompliance Related to Medical Treatment.
    4. Body Image, Disturbed Related to Acne.

16. A 4-year-old male client is visiting the pediatrician for papules and vesicles between his fingers. The physician takes a tongue blade and scrapes the area onto a slide. The mother asks the nurse, "What is he doing?" The best response by the nurse is:
    1. "The physician is trying to remove the irritant."
    2. "The physician is scraping the skin to determine if there are mites."
    3. "The physician is scraping the skin to remove dead skin layers."
    4. "The physician is removing a lesion."

17. A client has been diagnosed with scabies. What education should be provided for this client and his/her parents?
    1. Clean all carpets with a pesticide.
    2. Clean all clothing with mild detergent and use fabric softener.
    3. Clean all linen, clothing, towels, and washclothes with hot water and dry at a high heat.
    4. Clean the bedroom thoroughly to remove all dust mites.

CRITICAL THINKING EXERCISE

Read the case study. Answer the questions, keeping in mind the steps of the nursing process: assessing, diagnosing, planning, implementing, and evaluating.

A mother and her 15-year-old son are visiting the physician. The client has a lesion on his upper lip, which is a reddened, vesicle with yellowish, exudate. The physician informs the client that the lesion is caused by herpes. The physician leaves the room, and the mother and client are very upset.

1. What information should the nurse provide that might calm the client?
2. When is this lesion likely to occur?
3. How is it treated?
4. How long does it take to treat the lesion?

Chapter 25

Care of the Child with Endocrine Disorders

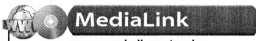

www.prenhall.com/towle

Use the address above to access the free, interactive Companion Website created for this textbook. Get hints, instant feedback to chapter-related NCLEX®-style questions. Link to other interesting sites.

Audio Glossary:

Use the Companion Website, or the CD-ROM disk enclosed with your textbook, to hear the pronunciation of key terms in the chapter.

The endocrine system communicates and controls many body systems by hormones that target certain organs. The secretion and inhibition of hormones occurs by positive and negative feedback system. Once blood levels of a hormone have reached the appropriate level, the negative feedback system signals the inhibition of the hormone. Contrary, the positive feedback system signals the release of a hormone in response to the increase another substance in the blood.

Endocrine disorders are difficult to detect. Detection of these disorders occurs by a process of elimination of disorders until a diagnosis is made. Once a diagnosis has been made, the process of treating the disorder may take time, as the endocrine system is a precise system and can be difficult to regulate.

This study guide chapter will allow the reader to understand hematological and lymphatic disorders that affect the pediatric client. Knowledge of hematological and lymphatic disorders and how they are medically managed will allow the student to apply the nursing process in managing the pediatric client with these disorders.

MATCHING

Match the term in the left column with the correct definition in the right column.

1. _____ Growth hormone   A.   Fat deposits on the back between the shoulder blades

2. _____ Parathyroid hormone   B.   Enlargement of the thyroid gland

3. _____ Epinephrine   C.   Glucose in the urine

4. _____ Galactosemia   D.   Excessive urination

5. _____ Tay–Sachs disease   E.   Hormone for normal growth

6. _____ Polyuria   F.   Diagnosed at age 3 to 6 months

7. _____ Goiter   G.   Antibodies attack the thyroid gland

8. _____ Grave's disease   H.   Adrenaline

9. _____ Buffalo hump
10. _____ Glucosuria

I. Inability to metabolize carbohydrates
J. Increases the amount of calcium in the blood

FILL IN THE BLANKS

Fill in the blanks with the appropriate word or phrase.

1. Without _____, water is not reabsorbed by the kidneys.

2. _____ is also called "bulging eyes."

3. _____ should be administered immediately for the client who has ketoacidosis.

4. A health promotion activity for the diabetic client involves inspecting the _____ daily for redness, swelling, or sores.

5. The _____ nurse may need to assist the client in monitoring glucose levels during the school day.

6. A female client with diabetes mellitus type 1 may experience _____ _____ when experiencing a state of hyperglycemia.

7. This type of diabetes mellitus type _____ is on the increase in the United States.

MULTIPLE CHOICE

Circle the answer that best completes the following statements.

1. You receive a 5-day-old male infant from the emergency department with a diagnosis of dehydration. During the admission assessment, you learn the client has had vomiting and diarrhea and is not eating well. The emergency department nurse reported a serum glucose of 60. You suspect:
   1. Diabetes insipidus.
   2. Diabetes mellitus.
   3. Galactosemia.
   4. Ketoacidosis.

2. The physician has ordered a nutrition consultation with a dietician for the infant diagnosed with maple syrup urine disease (MSUD). The mother asks why a consult with the dietician is necessary. An appropriate response would be:
   1. "A dietician can provide a well-balanced diet regimen for your child."
   2. "A dietician is consulted for every infant who is admitted to the pediatric unit."
   3. "A dietician is consulted to help you provide proper fluids to increase your son's urine output."
   4. "A dietician will develop a diet that will help you eliminate the amino acids your son should not receive."

FILL IN THE BLANKS

Fill in the blanks with the appropriate word or phrase.

1. This acronym, A _____, B _____,
   C _____ , D _____, and E _____,
   is useful when inspecting a suspicious lesion or mole.
2. _____ is inflammation of the skin.
3. _____ is a chronic inflammatory disorder of the skin.
4. A blackhead is also called a(n) _____.
5. _____ is freezing with liquid nitrogen.
6. _____ adds pigment or color to the skin.
7. A(n) _____ _____ is caused by some source
   of heat such as fire and hot liquids.

MULTIPLE CHOICE

Circle the answer that best completes the following statements.

1. A mother has brought her 3-month-old infant into the pediatrician's office for
   a rash. Upon examination, the nurse notes vesicles and papules on the infant's
   extremities and trunk. The pediatrician diagnosis miliaria and informs the
   nurse to provide instructions to the mother. What information should the
   nurse include in her instructions?
   1. Encourage fluids, provide a quiet environment, and Tylenol prn for a
      temperature of 101°F or greater.
   2. Provide a cool environment; avoid humidity, offer cool baths and med-
      icated powder prn for itching.
   3. Provide calming music, offer warm baths, and Benadryl prn for itching.
   4. Offer warm baths, force fluids and Tylenol prn for fussiness.

2. An 18-month-old female is admitted for cellulitis of the axilla and groin. Upon
   admission, the nurse notes redness, moisture, and a whitish-thick substance in
   the axilla and groin areas. This client is large, and her brachial and thigh areas
   appear to cause friction of these areas upon movement. The nurse suspects:
   1. Impetigo.
   2. Thrush.
   3. Intertrigo.
   4. Strawberry mark.

3. A father brings his 4-year-old son into the pediatrician's office for a rash on
   his extremities. The rash is reddened and has vesicles. The father states, "We
   were in the woods last weekend, and I think its poison ivy." The pediatrician
   examines the rash, diagnoses contact dermatitis, and informs the father he will
   write a prescription for a topical cream to be applied to the area. The father

asks the nurse, "What is contact dermatitis? I thought it was poison ivy." The most appropriate response by the nurse would be:

1. "Contact dermatitis is a medical term that means an irritant has caused a rash. Poison ivy can cause this condition."
2. "I'll have the pediatrician explain his diagnosis."
3. "Contact dermatitis means someone has transmitted this rash to your son."
4. "This is a rash that will clear up once you've used the medication for a few days."

4. You are working in a well-child clinic. The pediatric nurse practitioner diagnoses contact dermatitis in the groin area of a 2-year-old client and asks you to educate the mother on methods she may take at home to help prevent this condition in the future. Which of the following topics should you include in your education?

1. Warm baths, cool environment, and encourage fluids.
2. Keeping the groin area clean, dry and allowing air and light to the area.
3. Keeping the groin area clean and changing clothing often.
4. Encouraging fluids, bubble baths, and clean clothes.

5. A neighbor brings her 6-month-old son over to your house because she knows you are a nurse and wants your advice. She states, "My son has diaper rash, and I don't know what to do." Which of the following statements offers the best advice for this mother?

1. "You should call your physician."
2. "Keep the area clean and dry. Use absorbent diapers, wash his groin and anus with warm soap and water, dry the area, and apply a diaper-rash ointment."
3. "Keep the area clean and dry. Call your pediatrician if it doesn't clear up in a few days."
4. "Just change his diapers often; it will clear up in a few days."

6. The same neighbor in question #5 shows you her son's scalp. He has an area of dried, yellow patches on the frontal area of his scalp. The neighbor asks, "What do you think this is?" Which of the following conditions would you suspect?

1. Lice
2. Contact dermatitis
3. Seborrheic dermatitis
4. Scabies

7. A nurse practitioner informs a mother her son has "cradle cap." The nurse practitioner instructs you to educate the mother on how to manage this condition at home. What instructions do you provide for this mother?

1. Cleanse the area every day and wear a hat when outdoors.
2. Apply an emollient to the area and remove the debris.
3. Cleanse the area with a dandruff shampoo.
4. Apply an emollient to the area and remove debris; wash the scalp with baby shampoo.

3. A mother with a 9-month-old infant is visiting the pediatrician for a well-child visit. The infant was recently diagnosed with Tay–Sachs disease. The mother informs the nurse that she would like to become pregnant in a few months but is concerned about having another child with this disease. The nurse should:
   1. inform the mother Tay–Sachs is a genetic disease that can be detected through genetic counseling.
   2. inform the mother of a clinic that specializes with Tay–Sachs disease.
   3. call the office manager into the room so she may inform the mother of the proper actions to take.
   4. refer the mother to an obstetrician.

4. You are caring for a 9-year-old male client who is admitted with a diagnosis of diabetes insipidus. When obtaining a health history which of the following would correlate to this diagnosis?
   1. A history of meningitis.
   2. A history of diabetes mellitus.
   3. A history of an automobile accident.
   4. A deficiency of growth hormone during infancy.

5. A school-age client has been diagnosed with diabetes insipidus. The nurse advises the mother to contact the school regarding:
   1. The ability to eat whenever the child thinks his blood glucose is low.
   2. The ability to go to the bathroom whenever necessary.
   3. The freedom to call his mother whenever he deems necessary.
   4. The psychological issues of the client's disease.

6. A 12-year-old male is visiting the physician due to his inability to sleep. The nurse is obtaining a set of vital signs, notices exophthalmos, obtains a recent history, and learns the client has been failing at school. The mother states, "He doesn't seem to hear me. I have to tell him several times to do his chores." The nurse suspects the client has:
   1. Graves' disease.
   2. Diabetes insipidus.
   3. Hypothyroidism.
   4. Hyperthyroidism.

7. A client with a history of asthma for 10 years has presented to the pediatrician's office with the following symptoms: rounded cheeks, double chin, buffalo hump, and weight gain. The nurse suspects:
   1. Hypopituitarism.
   2. Hyperpituitarism.
   3. Cushing's syndrome.
   4. ADH.

8. A 10-year-old male client is admitted with a diagnosis of "hypertension, unknown etiology." Upon admission, the client complains of severe headache, weakness, increased thirst, and a blood pressure of 184/96. The nurse suspects:
   1. Cushing's syndrome.
   2. Diabetes mellitus.
   3. Adrenal insufficiency.
   4. Pheochromocytoma.

9. A 12-year-old male client and his father are visiting a surgeon to have an adrenal gland removed for pheochromocytoma. The surgeon informs the client and his father that a 24-hour urine will be obtained a few days postop. The father is frustrated and states, "We've already done this test. Why do we have to repeat this test?" The most appropriate response by the nurse is:
   1. "A 24-hour urine is done to ensure the kidneys are functioning properly."
   2. "A 24-hour urine is done to ensure the entire tumor has been removed and everything is fine."
   3. "This test is required postoperatively by your insurance."
   4. "This must be done to ensure your child has not developed complications from this surgery."

10. A client reports he is feeling shaky, weak, and dizzy. When you talk with him, he becomes easily irritated and says, "I haven't eaten all day. I'm so hungry I could eat a horse. Get me something to eat!" From these assessment data, which of the following interventions would be most appropriate?
    1. Check the client's blood sugar and provide a snack.
    2. Have the client lie down and administer oxygen.
    3. Monitor the client for orthostatic hypotension.
    4. Call the physician for an order for an IV.

11. When caring for a client with pheochromocytoma, the nurse must:
    1. Monitor blood glucose.
    2. Administer oxygen.
    3. Monitor blood pressure.
    4. Assess for signs of infection.

12. Which of the following disorders occurs when the adrenal glands do not secrete enough corticosteroids?
    1. Addison's disease.
    2. Cushing's syndrome.
    3. Pheochromocytoma.
    4. Thyroid toxicosis.

13. Which of the following symptoms would be consistent with a diagnosis of Cushing's disease?
    1. Bronze color of the skin; hypotension
    2. Pounding headache; diaphoresis
    3. Increased glucose levels; fatty tissue deposits
    4. Intolerance to cold; lethargy

14. You are caring for a pediatric client with a diagnosis of weakness and dehydration. You review the following serum lab results of sodium 128, glucose 65, and potassium 4.9. You suspect:
    1. Pheochromocytoma.
    2. Addison's disease.
    3. Cushing's syndrome.
    4. Diabetes insipidus.

15. A 15-year-old client is admitted with a medical diagnosis of "rule out urinary tract infection." While obtaining information during the admission process, you learn the client has had increased urination, increased thirst, and hunger. You suspect:
    1. Diabetes insipidus.
    2. Hypothyroidism.
    3. Hyperthyroidism.
    4. Diabetes mellitus.

16. You are working in the emergency department and receive a 14-year-old female who presents with the following signs and symptoms: fruity breath, decreased level of consciousness, and facial flushing. You suspect:
    1. Hyperglycemia.
    2. Hydronephrosis.
    3. Diabetic ketoacidosis.
    4. Pyelonephrosis.

17. You receive a client with a diagnosis of diabetic ketoacidosis. Which IV solution should be administered?
    1. D5W.
    2. Normal saline.
    3. Half-strength normal saline.
    4. Lactated Ringer's.

CRITICAL THINKING EXERCISE

Read the case study. Answer the questions, keeping in mind the steps of the nursing process: assessing, diagnosing, planning, implementing, and evaluating.

You are working in the emergency department when a 12-year-old client arrives with the following signs and symptoms: fruity breath, flushing of skin, Kussmaul's respirations, serum potassium of 5.5, and decreased level of consciousness.

1. What is your first action?
2. What is your next action?
3. What type of IV solution should be initiated?
4. Once urine output is established, what should be administered IV?
5. Once IV potassium is administered, what should the nurse monitor?

Chapter 26

Care of the Child with a Communicable Disease

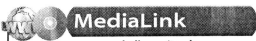

Communicable diseases are transmitted from one person to another by way of direct contact with body fluids or indirectly such as through contact with contaminated objects. Diseases can spread easily between pediatric clients by both direct and indirect contact.

The nurse has an important role in recognizing these diseases and assisting the family in obtaining appropriate care. Communicable diseases can be prevented in many cases. Another important nursing role is client and family teaching regarding methods of disease prevention.

This study guide chapter will allow the reader to understand communicable diseases that affect the pediatric client. Knowledge of communicable disorders and how they are medically managed will allow the student to apply the nursing process in managing the pediatric client with these disorders.

MATCHING

Match the term in the left column with the correct definition in the right column.

1. _____ Reverse isolation   A. Precautions to protect from body fluids

2. _____ Lyme disease   B. Inanimate object

3. _____ Rabies   C. Period prior to onset of symptoms

4. _____ Erythema migrans   D. Protects client from harmful organisms

5. _____ Immunization   E. A harmful organism

6. _____ Standard Precautions   F. Transmitted by a tick

7. _____ Prodromal period   G. Period of pathogen transmission to onset of symptoms

8. _____ Incubation period   H. Caused by Rhabdoviridae virus

9. _____ Fomite

I.   Administered parenterally to induce immunity

10. _____ Pathogen

J.   Red rash with a bull's-eye appearance

FILL IN THE BLANKS

Fill in the blanks with the appropriate word or phrase.

1. _____ _____ _____ is a release of deadly infectious agents for the purpose of causing chaos and fear.

2. _____ may be transmitted prenatally or a birth.

3. The _____ period is the time from the transmission of the pathogen and the onset of symptoms.

4. A(n) _____ is an inanimate object.

5. The _____ _____ _____ is the transmission in which the harmful organism enters a new host.

MULTIPLE CHOICE

Circle the answer that best completes the following statements.

1. You are working at a well-child clinic during the summer months. The nurse practitioner asks you to educate a mother on method she may utilize to decrease her son's risk of obtaining Lyme disease. Which of the following would be appropriate?
   1. Use of oil-based lotions to deter insects.
   2. Use of insect repellant.
   3. Wearing light colored clothing.
   4. Avoiding the evening hours.

2. You receive a 7-year-old client with a diagnosis of possible rabies. What type of protective equipment should you place outside the client's room?
   1. Gown, gloves, and mask.
   2. Gloves and mask.
   3. Gloves.
   4. Gown and gloves.

3. You are working in a pediatrician's office, and the mother of a 6-year-old female who was recently diagnosed with chickenpox is on the phone. She states she is having difficulty keeping her daughter from scratching her lesions. What would you recommend?
   1. Hot compresses and a dose of Benadryl.
   2. Cool compresses, calamine lotion, and distraction activities.
   3. Distraction activities and aspirin as needed.
   4. Aspirin and calamine lotion.

4. You are caring for a pediatric client who is admitted with cellulitis secondary to chickenpox. An appropriate nursing intervention would be:
   1. Application of ice to pulse points.
   2. Application of a dressing to the area.
   3. Trimming fingernails.
   4. Application of lotion to the area.

5. You are caring for a client with a diagnosis of "rule out Reye's syndrome." The client is crying and very irritable. The mother states, "Can't you give her some aspirin?" An appropriate response would be:
   1. "I will get some Tylenol because aspirin is contraindicated for Reye's syndrome."
   2. "I need to obtain a set of vital signs and then I will get the aspirin."
   3. "Your daughter needs to be distracted. I'll get a video for her to watch."
   4. "Why do you think your daughter needs aspirin?"

6. A mother has a child with a diagnosis of chickenpox. The mother asks the nurse what measures she can take at home to prevent the transmission of the virus to her other children. Which would be an appropriate action?
   1. Isolate the other children from the contagious child.
   2. Force fluids and require complete bed rest of all children.
   3. Require frequent handwashing for everyone in the household.
   4. Empty the trash from the home that contains contaminated tissues.

7. A pediatric client who has received chemotherapy is placed in reverse isolation. The mother states she does not understand why she must wear a mask and gown when around her son. Which would be an accurate rationale?
   1. Reverse isolation is designed to protect the client from the transmission of organisms.
   2. Reverse isolation is for those individuals who have contagious illnesses.
   3. The mother does not understand that reverse isolation is to protect her from her son's harmful organisms.
   4. Reverse isolation is a proactive action to ensure no organisms are transmitted to the client and/or visitor.

8. Which of the following clients should be placed in reverse isolation?
   1. Those who have highly contagious illnesses.
   2. Those who are positive for HIV.
   3. Those who are immunosuppressed.
   4. Those who have a WBC of 6,000.

9. You are caring for a 9-year-old male client with a medical diagnosis of Rocky Mountain spotted fever. You notice bleeding of the client's gums after he has brushed his teeth. What is your concern regarding this symptom?
   1. Gingivitis.
   2. Thrush.
   3. Herpes simplex type 1.
   4. GI and/or other bleeding.

10. You are educating parents at a local community event about the transmission of Lyme disease and Rocky Mountain spotted fever. Which of the following are important actions to include?
    1. Wear light-colored clothing when outdoors.
    2. Limit time outdoors to 2 hours per day in the summer.
    3. Use an insect repellant that contains DEET.
    4. Apply emollient lotions to prevent adherence of ticks to the skin.

11. A 7-year-old female client enters the emergency department after receiving a dog bite. Which action should the nurse perform first?
    1. Obtain a temperature.
    2. Obtain a urinalysis.
    3. Obtain a CBC.
    4. Wash the wound with warm soap and water.

12. You are caring for a client who is receiving several doses of corticosteroids for exacerbation of asthma. Which of the following nursing diagnoses would be appropriate for this client?
    1. Developmental Delay, Risk for Related to Chronic Illness
    2. Infection, Risk for Related to Medication Regimen
    3. Health Maintenance, Ineffective Related to Chronic Illness
    4. Memory, Impaired Related to Medication Regimen

13. You are caring for a client who is in contact isolation. The client's mother asks the nurse why her daughter has her own stethoscope and thermometer. An appropriate response would be:
    1. "Everyone has their own stethoscope and thermometer."
    2. "Because she's in isolation."
    3. "Items that come in contact with your daughter may transmit her illness to others; for this reason she has her own equipment."
    4. "Someone must have left these in here. I'll remove them."

14. A mother has her 3-year-old son in the pediatrician's office for a well-child visit. The nurse takes the client's temperature and obtains a reading of 100.2°F. The mother informs the pediatrician her son has been irritable and not sleeping well. The pediatrician, mumbles, "It may be the prodromal period of the flu." The mother asks the nurse what this term means. An appropriate response would be:
    1. "It means your son is contagious."
    2. "It means the beginning vague symptoms of an illness."
    3. "It means we must isolate your son from others."
    4. "It means your son is displaying signs and symptoms that are benign."

15. You are training another LPN/LVN nurse in the pediatrician's office. The nurse asks you which type of immunity immunizations provide:
    1. Passive immunity.
    2. Active immunity.
    3. Natural immunity.
    4. Acquired immunity.

16. A pediatric client is placed in droplet isolation. This type of isolation is provided because:
    1. This isolation is to protect those who are within 3 feet of the client.
    2. This isolation is to protect those from inhaling the pathogens.
    3. This type of isolation is to protect others from fomites, which may contain the pathogen.
    4. This isolation is for all direct admissions that have a temperature greater than 101°F.

17. You are working in a pediatrician's office. The pediatrician orders the client receive immunotherapy for her allergies. The mother asks, "What is immunotherapy?" An appropriate response would be:
    1. "It is a process in which we expose your child to the allergen."
    2. "It is a process in which we inject a small amount of the allergens, and over time your daughter will build up her immunity."
    3. "It is a process in which large amounts of various allergens are injected, and your daughter's immune system becomes resistant."
    4. "A sample of your daughter's blood is sent to be analyzed and a vaccine is developed."

CRITICAL THINKING EXERCISE

Read the case study. Answer the questions, keeping in mind the steps of the nursing process: assessing, diagnosing, planning, implementing, and evaluating.

You are caring for a 4-year-old female client of Asian decent. The child is admitted with a diagnosis of dehydration secondary to influenza. An IV of D5½ NS at 50 mL per hour has been initiated. The physician has ordered clear liquids and bed rest. You are performing your shift assessment and notice circular bruising near the scapular areas and midposterior thorax area.

1. What additional information would you obtain from the parents?
2. Do the parents practice cultural therapies?
3. What would you want to rule out?
4. What other information would you want to know about cupping?
5. How do you manage this family's cultural beliefs?

Chapter 27

Care of the Child with Psychosocial Disorders

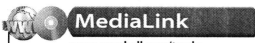
MediaLink
www.prenhall.com/towle

Use the address above to access the free, interactive Companion Website created for this textbook. Get hints, instant feedback to chapter-related NCLEX®-style questions. Link to other interesting sites.

Audio Glossary:

Use the Companion Website, or the CD-ROM disk enclosed with your textbook, to hear the pronunciation of key terms in the chapter.

Psychosocial health is comprised of emotional, spiritual, social, and mental well-being. Children who are emotionally, socially, mentally, and spiritually healthy have the ability to manage life's stressors, make good decisions, and manage social situations. A child's psychosocial health is affected by many factors—financial status, genetics, self-esteem, family, physical health, and cultural beliefs.

This study guide chapter will allow the reader to understand psychosocial disorders that affect the pediatric client. Knowledge of psychosocial disorders and how they are medically managed will allow the student to apply the nursing process in managing the pediatric client with these disorders.

MATCHING

Match the term in the left column with the correct definition in the right column.

1. _____ Stereotypy
2. _____ Echolalia
3. _____ Encopresis
4. _____ GAD
5. _____ Copropraxia
6. _____ OCD
7. _____ Tics
8. _____ Bipolar disorder
9. _____ Bulimia
10. _____ Purging

A. Generalized anxiety disorder
B. Sudden, rapid motor movements
C. Involuntary obscene gesture
D. Self-induced vomiting
E. Repeating words
F. Rigid and obsessive behaviors
G. Delayed defecation
H. Binge eating and purging
I. Disorder of severe mood swings
J. Obsessive-compulsive disorder

FILL IN THE BLANKS

Fill in the blanks with the appropriate word or phrase.

1. A suicidal thought is _____.
2. The _____ is the diagnostic tool utilized by mental health professionals in the United States.
3. This syndrome, _____, usually has a later onset than autism.
4. In _____ _____, pediatric clients may voice obscenities, use racial slurs, and display obscene gestures.
5. The nurse must report to state and local authorities any suspicion of _____ _____.
6. A nurse may lose his/her _____ if he/she fails to report abuse.
7. _____ is a form of emotional and physical abuse.

MULTIPLE CHOICE

Circle the answer that best completes the following statements.

1. Your 11-year-old daughter's best friend has been displaying mood swings. The child's mother asks your advice. She states, "I don't know what to do. One week she's extremely happy, and the next week she's very depressed." You suspect this child may have:
    1. Generalized anxiety disorder.
    2. Obsessive-compulsive disorder.
    3. Separation anxiety disorder.
    4. Bipolar disorder.
2. The mother in question #1 asks you, "What should I do?" Which of the following would be an appropriate response?
    1. "You should admit her to a psychiatric facility for evaluation."
    2. "I would make an appointment with your pediatrician and inform him/her of your concerns."
    3. "I would make an appointment with a psychologist."
    4. "I would take her to the emergency department now."
3. You are working in a pediatrician's office and are taking vital signs on a 3-year-old client. The client allows you to touch him without hesitation or fear. The mother states her son has been repeating words successively and frequently and rocking while repeating these words. You suspect this client may have:
    1. Obsessive-compulsive disorder.
    2. Generalized anxiety disorder.
    3. Autism.
    4. Separation anxiety disorder.

4. The pediatrician assesses the client in question #3 and comments, "He's displaying echolalia." The mother asks you what this term means. An appropriate response would be:
    1. "It means your son is repeating words frequently."
    2. "It means he has a medical condition that can be treated with medication."
    3. "It means your son is very intelligent."
    4. "It's just a medical term that indicates a change in one's speech patterns."

5. (Same scenario as in question 3.) The physician orders an MRI. The mother asks the nurse, "Why does he want to perform an MRI on my child?" The best response would be:
    1. "I'm not sure. I'll have the doctor explain it to you."
    2. "It is done routinely for children who display changes in their speech patterns."
    3. "It is done to rule out any other cause for the symptoms your son is displaying."
    4. "It's done because the doctor has his reasons."

6. You are working in a pediatrician's office and ask the mother of a 6-year-old male client what the reason is for their visit. The mother states that her son is easily distracted, has difficulty working with others, and has difficulty completing assignments in school. She states that her son's teacher recommended an examination by the pediatrician. You suspect the teacher believes the client may have:
    1. Generalized anxiety disorder.
    2. Autism.
    3. Attention deficit disorder.
    4. School phobia.

7. A psychologist is providing a community education fair for pediatric psychosocial issues. The psychologist informs a parent their child may have *anaclitic depression*. You understand another term for this is:
    1. Separation anxiety disorder.
    2. Generalized anxiety disorder.
    3. Depression.
    4. School phobia.

8. A mother has brought her 9-year-old daughter to be seen by the pediatrician because of anxiety. The mother informs the pediatrician that her daughter worries obsessively about possible issues that may or may not arise in the future. You suspect the client has:
    1. Obsessive-compulsive disorder.
    2. Anxiety.
    3. Generalized anxiety disorder.
    4. Attention deficit hyperactivity disorder.

9. The major cause of death among adolescents is:
    1. Suicide.
    2. Cancer.
    3. Poisoning.
    4. Injuries.

10. A 16-year-old client tells the nurse, "I just want to die. I have nothing to live for." The nurse's best response would be:
    1. "Oh, stop that kind of talk. You've got everything to live for."
    2. "It is best to think positive thoughts rather than to be so negative."
    3. "I think you're trying to get attention from your parents."
    4. "You sound very sad. Let's sit down and talk about your feelings."

11. You are talking to a 14-year-old female client who has been using the tip of a metal nail file to inflict superficial cuts on her body. Which of the following activities might be helpful for this client when she feels compelled to engage in the self-injurious behavior?
    1. Write in a journal.
    2. Call a friend who also cuts.
    3. Eat a piece of chocolate.
    4. Smoke a cigarette.

12. You are working as a school nurse in a local high school. A teacher asks you to come to her class and examine a 16-year-old male who is exhibiting drowsiness. You assess dilated pupils, drowsiness, and extreme mood swings. You suspect:
    1. Postictal seizure.
    2. Drug abuse.
    3. Cigarette abuse.
    4. Dysfunctional family situation.

13. A 10-day-old newborn is admitted to the pediatric unit for "failure to thrive." You observe fussiness and poor eating. You suspect:
    1. Nonorganic failure to thrive.
    2. Failure to thrive related to poor eating.
    3. Fetal alcohol syndrome.
    4. Shaken baby syndrome.

14. A child who has experienced a traumatic event needs which of the following?
    1. Frequent touching, communication regarding the specifics of the event and time alone.
    2. Love, reassurance, frequent cuddling, and the ability to ask questions and receive honest answers to their questions.
    3. Love, reassurance, and the ability to answer and receive answers to their questions.
    4. Reassurance and honest answers to their questions.

15. A pediatric client is recently diagnosed with autism. The pediatrician informs the client's father he is going to prescribe a medication for the client. The father asks the nurse, "What kind of medication will he prescribe?" You suspect the pediatrician will prescribe:
    1. Antipsychotic medication.
    2. Tricyclic medication.
    3. Serotonin reuptake inhibitor.
    4. Beta-blocker medication.

16. You are caring for a 5-year-old male client with a diagnosis of autism. The client is admitted to the pediatric unit with gastroenteritis. The child is frustrated and banging his head on the wall when you enter the room. An appropriate nursing intervention would be:
    1. Physically remove the client from the wall.
    2. Go and order a helmet from central supply.
    3. Go to the medication cart and draw up a sedative to administer stat.
    4. Call for help.

17. You are working in the emergency department and receive a 15-year-old female client who is emaciated, bradycardic, and depressed. Her friends brought her in because she had a syncopal episode at the mall. You suspect this client has:
    1. Bulimia.
    2. Obsessive-compulsive disorder.
    3. Depression.
    4. Anorexia nervosa.

18. You are caring for a 17-year-old female client who was admitted with a diagnosis of syncope and electrolyte imbalance. You are performing a shift assessment and notice the enamel is off some of her teeth. You suspect:
    1. Anorexia nervosa.
    2. Bulimia.
    3. Depression.
    4. Binging disorder.

CRITICAL THINKING EXERCISE

Read the case study. Answer the questions, keeping in mind the steps of the nursing process: assessing, diagnosing, planning, implementing, and evaluating.

You are caring for a 9-year-old female client on the pediatric unit with a medical diagnosis of recurrent urinary tract infections. The client is withdrawn when asked questions and appears fearful of staff. The mother informs you her daughter is complaining of burning and itching in the perineal area. You inform the mother and the client you need to examine her perineum. You notice bruising and redness on the client's labia majora and minora.

1. What information would you want to obtain from the client?
2. If the client indicates she has been sexually abused, which action should you take next?
3. How do you handle the mother in this situation?
4. Who should be contacted in regard to the client?

Chapter 28

Care of the Family with a Dying Child

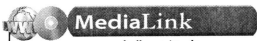

MediaLink

www.prenhall.com/towle

Use the address above to access the free, interactive Companion Website created for this textbook. Get hints, instant feedback to chapter-related NCLEX®-style questions. Link to other interesting sites.

Audio Glossary:

Use the Companion Website, or the CD-ROM disk enclosed with your textbook, to hear the pronunciation of key terms in the chapter.

The death of a child may be expected after a chronic illness or unexpected such as a result of an injury. Parents and siblings involved in the care of a chronically ill child may have a sense of involvement in the death process of the deceased. On the contrary, parents and siblings who loose a child suddenly may have difficulty coping with the loss of their loved one.

Five stages of loss or grief have been identified through research. This study guide chapter will allow the reader to understand the grief or loss process that affects the pediatric client's family. Knowledge of psychological issues surrounding death and how they affect the family will allow the student to apply the nursing process in assisting the family who is experiencing the death of a child.

MATCHING

Match the term in the left column with the correct definition in the right column.

1. _____ Dysfunctional grief

2. _____ Palliative care

3. _____ Euthanasia

4. _____ Mottled

5. _____ Cheyne–Stokes breathing

6. _____ Autopsy

7. _____ Loss

8. _____ Grief

A. Periods of deep breathing followed by periods of apnea

B. Extreme sadness

C. Examination of the body after death

D. Palliative care focused on quality of life and not a cure

E. Something is removed

F. Stiffening of the body after death

G. One who is unable to accept what has happened and move on with their life

H. Care is focused on relief from suffering

9. _____ Hospice care
10. _____ Rigor mortis

I.   Compassionately putting someone to death
J.   Purplish marbled appearance

FILL IN THE BLANKS

Fill in the blanks with the appropriate word or phrase.

1. When caring for a child with a chronic terminal illness, parents have more
    _____ to prepare for the loss.

2. As a grandparent grieves for the loss of a grandchild and the pain their adult
    child is experiencing, their _____ may go unnoticed or unmet.

3. By communicating _____, the nurse may assist the grand-
    parent in dealing with their loss.

4. A client must be _____ _____ before organ
    donation may take place.

5. The family must move past their _____ and _____
    before they can be approached about possible organ donation.

6. The preschool client believes death is _____.

7. A client with a(n) _____ _____ and in
    critical condition should be considered for potential organ donation.

MULTIPLE CHOICE

Circle the answer that best completes the following statements.

1. A 17-year-old client with a diagnosis of muscular dystrophy has recently ex-
    pired. The father of the child comments, "I feel guilty for being happy about
    his death. He is no longer suffering." The most appropriate response by the
    nurse is:
    1. "It is okay to feel guilty; all parents do when something happens to
        their child."
    2. "Would you like to talk about it?"
    3. "Why do you feel guilty?"
    4. "Why are you happy about his death?"

2. A 7-year-old sibling of a client who is dying is sitting in the pediatric playroom
    and appears sad. The parents of the client are busy caring for the child. The
    nurse can assist the sibling in dealing with his/her sadness at this time by:
    1. having the sibling color a picture or make a card for the client.
    2. having the sibling express his/her feelings toward the dying client.
    3. having a parent come into the playroom and assist the child.
    4. calling a grandparent to take the child home.

3. A grandparent who experiences the loss of a grandchild may experience:
   1. Guilt and anger.
   2. Anger and intense grief.
   3. Guilt and hopelessness.
   4. Hopelessness and extreme sadness.

4. You are caring for a client whose parents have recently immigrated from India. The client is dying, and the nurse must approach the parents about funeral arrangements. As a nurse who is very knowledgeable about different cultures, you believe the parents will request:
   1. An autopsy.
   2. Cremation.
   3. A typical American funeral.
   4. Organ donation.

5. A pediatric client who was admitted with a medical diagnosis of dehydration has died suddenly. The family's religious beliefs are Jehovah's Witness. The pediatrician has recommended an autopsy. What do you expect the parent's reaction to be?
   1. Agree to an autopsy.
   2. Agree to a partial autopsy.
   3. Refuse until organs are harvested.
   4. Refuse because it is against their religious beliefs.

6. A family of the Muslim culture has just lost a female child. You notice several females entering the client's room with basins, towels, and linens. You suspect:
   1. They are bathing the client.
   2. They are bathing the client and preparing the body for burial.
   3. They are performing last rites on the client's body.
   4. They are performing a cleansing ritual.

7. A pediatric client with a terminal illness is dying. The client's parents have left the room for a few minutes. The nurse enters the room, and the child states, "I know I'm dying. What will happen to me?" The most appropriate response by the nurse would be:
   1. "Why do you think you're dying?"
   2. "What do you think will happen to you?"
   3. "Would you like to talk about your death?"
   4. "You're not dying, you're just ill."

8. A client with a terminal illness has had a change in condition. The nurse approaches the client and the family to discuss resuscitation orders and palliative care. The client states, "What is palliative care?" An appropriate response would be:
   1. "Palliative care does not cure you but makes you comfortable."
   2. "Palliative care provides some hope for a few clients and is experimental."
   3. "Palliative care provides extra nutrition when necessary."
   4. "Palliative care is when we insert a feeding tube when you are unable to eat."

9. You are working in the pediatric intensive care unit. A coworker asks you to notify an organ procurement organization (OPO), as a client is near death. You realize this is a:
   1. Hospital policy.
   2. State regulation.
   3. Federal policy.
   4. Cultural practice.

10. A mother is approached about donation of her daughter's organs. The mother states, "I can't afford to pay for that type of surgery." An appropriate response to the mother would be:
    1. "The family who receives the organ bears the expense."
    2. "The organ procurement organization bears the expense."
    3. "The hospital will bear the expense."
    4. "You can make payment arrangements with the hospital."

11. A mother of a 2-year-old child and a 7-year-old client who is dying are visiting the client. The 2-year-old is clinging to his mother. The mother states, "Since his brother has been very sick, he has been clinging to me. He even wants to sleep with me at night." The nurse identifies this behavior as:
    1. Generalized anxiety disorder.
    2. Depression.
    3. Regression.
    4. Separation anxiety disorder.

12. A mother who has recently lost a child is bringing her infant into the pediatrician for a well-child visit. The mother informs the nurse that since the death of her son, her infant daughter has been very fussy, is not eating well, and is not sleeping at night. The nurse realizes:
    1. The infant may be relating to the stress her mother is experiencing.
    2. The infant may have pyloric stenosis.
    3. The infant may have "failure to thrive."
    4. This is the method the infant exhibits their grief.

13. When answering a client's questions concerning his/her illness and impending death, it's best to:
    1. Avoid talking about it.
    2. Inform the parents so they may discuss it with their child.
    3. Be honest and speak in terms the client can understand.
    4. Ask the hospital social worker to speak with the client.

14. To stabilize a client who has passed for organ donation, what types of measures will be instituted?
    1. Maintaining cardiac output, monitoring electrolyte balance and proper ventilation and perfusion.
    2. Maintaining ventilation and cardiac monitoring.
    3. Maintaining cardiac and renal perfusion along with ventilator assistance.
    4. Ventilation assistance and maintaining cardiac perfusion.

15. Parents from Jamaica inform the nurse a "shaman" will visit their daughter tomorrow. The best response by the nurse is to:
    1. inform the parent they are in America and a shaman's practice would not be recognized.
    2. refuse to allow the shaman to visit the client.
    3. obtain more information.
    4. call the pediatrician and inform him/her of the parent's request.

16. A 5-year-old female client who is dying appears withdrawn. The nurse is concerned about communicating with the client. Which method would be likely to assist with communication?
    1. Obtain a doll or puppet so it may be utilized as a tool to promote communication.
    2. Obtain a graphic of a child of similar age and discuss the child in the graphic.
    3. Obtain crayons and a coloring book and color with the client hoping this will stimulate conversation.
    4. Communicate with the client via the parents.

CRITICAL THINKING EXERCISE

Read the case study. Answer the questions, keeping in mind the steps of the nursing process: assessing, diagnosing, planning, implementing, and evaluating.

You are caring for a client with a diagnosis of terminal cancer. The client is experiencing pain in both thighs. The mother requests more pain medication. The mother is upset because she requested her daughter receive more pain medication during the night and believes the nurse ignored her request.

1. What information would you want to obtain regarding the night shift nurse?
2. What action should you take regarding this situation?
3. What other comfort measures might assist in managing the client's pain?
4. What nursing diagnoses would be appropriate for this client?

Answer Key

Chapter 1 The LPN / LVN in Maternal-Child, Community-Based Nursing

Matching

1. E
2. H
3. A
4. D
5. F

6. I
7. C
8. J
9. G
10. B

Fill in the Blanks

1. pregnancy, childbirth, and postpartum
2. Association of Women's Health, Obstetrics, and Neonatal Nurses—AWHONN
3. pediatrics
4. interventions
5. Mortality
6. morbidity
7. cultural proficiency

Multiple Choice

1. 2, 3, 4
2. 3
3. 2
4. 2, 4, 3, 1
5. 3

6. 2
7. 1, 2, 4
8. 1
9. 3
10. 1

11. 3
12. 3
13. 1
14. 1
15. 4

Critical Thinking Exercise

1. The LPN/LVN may delegate tasks to the UAP. These tasks may include vital signs and assistance with ADLs.
2. No. Although the UAP is qualified to assist with ambulation, this client's ambulation experience will be used to provide an assessment of a condition. This is beyond the scope of practice for the UAP.
3. No. The UAP cannot delegate uncompleted tasks to another unlicensed person. The UAP must communicate inability to complete assignments to the LPN/LVN.
4. The LPN/LVN must first document their findings. Then, the physician's orders must be reviewed to determine the next course of action.

Chapter 2 Legal and Ethical Issues in Maternal-Child Nursing

Matching

1. D
2. C
3. A
4. F
5. H

6. E
7. G
8. I
9. B

Fill in the Blanks

1. *Healthy People 2000*
2. emancipated
3. Patient Self-Determination Act
4. assistive reproduction
5. right client, right drug, right dose, right route, right time
6. three (3)
7. WIC (Women, Infants, and Children)
8. the American Hospital Association
9. sexually transmitted infections, birth control, pregnancy, drug or alcohol treatment

Multiple Choice

1. 1
2. 3
3. 4
4. 4
5. 2

6. 3
7. 3, 4
8. 1, 3
9. 1
10. 4

11. 2
12. 2
13. 3
14. 2, 3, 4, 1
15. 3

Critical Thinking Exercise

1. Providing education concerning a procedure is the responsibility of the physician or health care professional performing the procedure.
2. The parent or guardian of the minor child has the responsibility for signing consent forms for treatments and procedures. The nurse may obtain the consents for the treatment/procedures.
3. There are situations/events that may negate the decision-making authority of parents/guardians. These situations may include

    If the parent (s) is (are) incapacitated and cannot make decisions

    If there is actual or suspected child abuse or neglect

    If the parent's choice does not permit lifesaving procedures for the child
4. The rights of the parents to make decisions may be affected if the treatments being refused are lifesaving in nature. Should lifesaving treatments be refused, the ethics committee of the health care facility will be consulted.
5. The role of the nurse is to ensure quality care to the client. When disparity exists between the nurse and the wishes of the parents, the nurse must put

their personal feelings aside. If the differences between the client, family, and nurse are significant or affecting the care, the nurse has the responsibility to notify the nursing supervisor.

6. Children do not have the right to refuse treatment. It is best, however, to keep children as involved as possible. Provide them age-appropriate information concerning the plan of care. Do not allow the child choices where none exist.

Chapter 3 Nursing Care of the Family

Matching

1.	D	6.	F
2.	G	7.	E
3.	C	8.	H
4.	B	9.	A
5.	J	10.	I

Fill in the Blanks

1. Family Development Theory
2. family-centered care
3. family
4. cult
5. culture
6. stereotyping
7. demandingness
8. ecomap
9. straight lines
10. the mother

Multiple Choice

1.	1, 3	7.	2	12.	4
2.	3	8.	1, 2	13.	3
3.	2	9.	1	14.	4
4.	3	10.	4	15.	1
5.	2	11.	1	16.	3, 4
6.	1, 2, 3				

Critical Thinking Exercise

1. The nurse will first need to review his or her own feelings about cultural diversity. The nurse will need to review knowledge of the traditions of both of the ethnic groups. It is important for the nurse to interact with each family unit in a respectful, individualized manner.

2. The American Black (African American) family is traditionally matriarchal. The extended family is of high importance in the American Black family. The

church is a source of social support. Access to primary health care may also be an issue.

3. There is no common language or religion with the Asian Pacific (Pacific Rim) group. The family is not time limited. The head of the household is typically the father. The household and childbearing responsibilities are left to the mother. Health care decisions are often up to the mother.

4. The nurse should begin by setting boundaries and must encourage each family to respect the privacy and space of the other. The nurse must be cognizant of privacy and confidentiality.

Chapter 4 Reproductive Anatomy and Physiology

Matching

1. D	6. H
2. B	7. J
3. G	8. A
4. I	9. C
5. E	10. F

Fill in the Blanks

1. chromosomes
2. adenine, thymine, guanine, and cystosine
3. vas deferens
4. 46
5. corpus luteum
6. rugae
7. Bartholin gland or greater vestibular glands
8. colostrum
9. menses, secretory, proliferative
10. excitement, plateau, orgasm, resolution

Multiple Choice

1. 1	6. 2	11. 3
2. 4	7. 2	12. 3
3. 3	8. 4	13. 1
4. 1, 3	9. 2	14. 2
5. 3	10. 1	15. 3, 4

Critical Thinking Exercise

1. The best time of the month to perform the self-breast examination is 5 days after the onset of menstruation. Consistency of day of the month will assist the examiner to be aware of cyclic related changes.

2. Hormones influence the size and sensitivity of breast tissue. Just prior to menstruation, the breast tissue is enlarged and tender. The levels of estrogen and progesterone are involved in these breast changes.

3. Positioning during the breast examination is important. The client should be instructed to position herself supine with a small towel under the shoulder. After completion of the examination, the client should observe the breast in four different positions. These positions include

   With arms relaxed at sides

   With arms lifted above the head

   With hands pressed against hips

   With hands pressed together at the waist and leaning forward.

   Some women may find showering an ideal time to perform the examination. If completed in the shower, the client should sit or stand with one hand behind the head.

4. The topic for the breast examination should be presented in a calm manner. Clients should feel comfortable asking questions. When the session is started, the nurse should provide guidelines and handouts. It may be useful for participants to be able to practice with models.

Chapter 5 Reproductive Issues

Matching Part I

1.	E	7.	J	13.	B
2.	H	8.	O	14.	M
3.	L	9.	A	15.	P
4.	Q	10.	K	16.	I
5.	G	11.	M	17.	D
6.	C	12.	F		

Matching Part II

1.	B	4.	E	
2.	C	5.	D	
3.	A	6.	C	

Fill in the Blanks

1. menopause
2. between the age of 35 and 58 years
3. location
4. thigh pain, hematuria, bloody stools, and anemia
5. inguinal
6. epididymitis
7. raw palmetto

Multiple Choice

1.	2	6.	3	11.	1, 2
2.	4	7.	3, 4	12.	4
3.	3	8.	1, 2, 4, 5	13.	3
4.	1	9.	2	14.	2
5.	3	10.	4	15.	4

Critical Thinking

1. The client diagnosed with cervical dysplasia will need information provided. The topics that should be included are

   The actual test results found

   Treatment options

   Prognosis

2. The risk factors associated with the development of cervical dysplasia include

   Infection by the human papilloma virus

   Early sexual intercourse

   HIV infection

   Smoking

   Poor diet

   Unprotected sex

   Multiple sexual partners

3. Cervical cell changes may be managed by laser treatments, cauterization, or conization.

4. Cervical dysplasia is seen as a precursor to the development of cervical cancer. Initially the cellular changes are *in situ*. Later, if these cells are left unchecked, the cancer will spread into surrounding tissues. Areas of spread include vaginal, urethra, bladder, and the rectum.

Chapter 6 Health Promotion During Pregnancy

Matching

1.	D	6.	L	11.	I
2.	G	7.	E	12.	C
3.	A	8.	O	13.	M
4.	J	9.	F	14.	B
5.	K	10.	H	15.	N

Fill in the Blanks

1. fallopian tubes
2. implantation

3. human chorionic gonadotropic hormone
4. glucose, proteins, urea, lanugo, vernix
5. the pre-embryonic state
6. umbilical vein
7. meconium
8. trimesters
9. chloasma

Multiple Choice

1.	4	6.	1, 2	11.	4
2.	1, 4, 5	7.	1	12.	3
3.	2	8.	2	13.	4
4.	1	9.	1	14.	2
5.	4	10.	1	15.	3

Critical Thinking Exercise

1. During the pregnancy, the body produces an increased amount of progesterone. Progesterone has smooth muscle relaxing properties. The muscular structures of the intestine are also relaxed. This results in a decrease in peristalsis. Physicians routinely prescribe prenatal vitamins containing iron. Iron has constipating side effects.
2. Diet, fluid intake, and activity can aid in management of constipation. Intake high in fiber is helpful to regulate the body's bowels. Fluid intake promotes positive elimination patterns.
3. The routine use of stool softeners is not typically recommended. To reduce dependence on medications the interventions listed in the previous response should be investigated.
4. Enema use is not recommended during pregnancy to manage constipation.

Chapter 7 Health Promotion During Labor and Delivery

Matching

1.	C	6.	G
2.	E	7.	A
3.	F	8.	I
4.	D	9.	J
5.	B	10.	H

Fill in the Blanks

1. Braxton Hicks contractions
2. bloody show
3. premature rupture of membranes
4. cephalopelvic disproportion
5. fetal lie

6. effleurage
7. latent
8. placental separation
9. Schultze mechanism
10. breech

Multiple Choice

1.	3	6.	2	11.	3
2.	1	7.	1, 3, 4	12.	4
3.	1	8.	2, 4	13.	3
4.	4	9.	2	14.	2
5.	2, 3	10.	3	15.	3

Critical Thinking Exercise

1. The epidural block will provide comfort during the labor process. The anesthesia will involve the lower abdomen, perineum, and lower legs. This will allow the client to remain awake and comfortable during the labor. The greatest disadvantages of the epidural relates to the potential decrease in participation in the labor process by the client. Some clients may have a reduced ability to push effectively, resulting in the need for increased assistance.

2. When caring for the client with an epidural the nurse must be aware of the potential side effects. These side effects include hypotension, bladder distention, and respiratory depression.

3. The use of general anesthesia for a vaginal delivery is not recommended. The medications used for general anesthesia can travel to the fetus in minutes and cause respiratory depression. In addition, the nurse should advise the client of the nursing care available to assist her in the management of her discomfort.

4. Systemic medications may be administered intravenously during active labor. These medications must be given only when the client's vital signs are within normal limits, the fetus is at term, and there is no fetal distress present.

Chapter 8 Maternal High-Risk Nursing Care

Matching

1.	G	6.	F
2.	J	7.	C
3.	B	8.	D
4.	E	9.	A
5.	I	10.	H

Fill in the Blanks

1. erythroblastosis fetalis
2. semi-Fowler's

3. fetal breathing, fetal movement, fetal tone, fluid volume, fetal reaction
4. dilation and curettage (D&C)
5. cerclage (also known as a Shirodkar procedure)
6. placenta previa
7. mild preeclampsia
8. retained placenta, uterine atony, lacerations

Multiple Choice

1.	2	6.	3	11.	2
2.	1, 2, 4	7.	2	12.	3
3.	2	8.	1	13.	3, 4, 1, 2
4.	3	9.	2	14.	1
5.	3, 4	10.	4	15.	4

Critical Thinking Exercise

1. Attempts should be made to assess fetal heart tones. An ultrasound is also indicated to assess for signs of fetal life.
2. If the fetus has died, it is termed a fetal demise or stillbirth.
3. The significant other or support person must be incorporated into the plan of care. The mother and family will be faced with numerous emotional hurdles in the event of the death of the baby. Efforts should be taken to include the significant other in the teaching and information being provided. The wishes of the client must be observed regarding privacy issues.
4. If the baby has died in utero, delivery will be based on a few factors. Labor may begin without initiation. If labor does not begin, the family may have the opportunity to return home and begin the grief process. Labor may be induced at a later date if the maternal condition does not contraindicate it.
5. The client will require the same physical care and assessments as a client who has delivered a living child. The emotional needs for this client will be significant. The client and her family should be allowed/encouraged to view and hold the baby. Photographs, footprints, and handprints should be recorded. If the client does not wish to take these photos home at the time of discharge, they should be kept of file for future requests. Information concerning support groups and other similar resources should be provided.

Chapter 9 Health Promotion of the Newborn

Matching

1.	G	6.	B
2.	F	7.	I
3.	H	8.	D
4.	J	9.	C
5.	A	10.	E

Fill in the Blanks

1. 500, 1000
2. Colostrum, yellow
3. lose
4. meconium, 24
5. on their back
6. bleeding
7. umbilical vein
8. cesarean section
9. 35, intraventricular hemorrhage
10. circumoral cyanosis

Multiple Choice

1. 1, 2, 3, 5
2. 1, 2, 3, 5
3. 4
4. 3
5. 4
6. 1
7. 3
8. 2
9. 2
10. 4
11. 2
12. 2
13. 3
14. 3
15. 2

Critical Thinking Exercise

1. This newborn has several concerns because it was delivered by emergency cesarean delivery (unplanned and did not proceed through the usual birthing process), is premature at 35 weeks gestation, is a first baby for the family, and has a congenital defect. Respiratory functioning is the highest priority. Thermoregulation, ability to nurse or bottle feed, and assessing for any other congenital problems are other priority areas.

2. The parents may be hesitant to be involved with any care with this newborn due to their emotional response to the cleft lip and palate and because of the prematurity. The newborn may need to be cared for in a special care nursery, which could further distance the parental involvement. Parents will need support during the adjustment period to and to possibly mourn the loss of their perfect child or delivery expectations. The mother will have her own recovery from surgery to experience. The nurse can assist and encourage the parents to be involved in much of the decision making regarding care, such as selection of assistive feeding products, changing of diapers, taking temperatures, keeping track of feeding frequency and volume (if bottle-fed, time nursed if breastfeeding), journaling thoughts and events as they occur.

3. Reviewing the mother's history to determine if there is anything that might be a continued influence on the newborn's health. Such findings may include extent of prenatal care, maternal drug or alcohol use, maternal health problems or medications, and blood type, including Rh factor. The presence of jaundice in the first 24 hours is very concerning. This rapid presence of jaundice is typically pathological jaundice in the newborn. This is due to an incompatibility of the Rh factor. If the mother has Rh negative blood and the newborn has Rh positive blood, this situation may result. This finding along with the presence of the jaundice would be critical to report to the charge

nurse and physician to make plans for the continued priority care of this newborn.

4. The situation has many problems and areas of teaching to consider: Long-term potential:
    1. Respiratory problems
    2. Discovery of other congenital defects
    3. Feeding problems
    4. Speech problems
    5. Infection after cleft lip/palate repair
    6. Parental bonding difficulties
    7. Risk for intraventricular hemorrhage
    8. Treatment of jaundice

Chapter 10 Health Promotion in the Postpartum Period

Matching

1.	C	6.	E
2.	J	7.	D
3.	B	8.	I
4.	A	9.	G
5.	H	10.	F

Fill in the Blanks

1. lochia
2. boggy
3. colostrum
4. postpartal chilling
5. engrossment
6. postpartum blues
7. positive Homan's sign
8. cold items—including food and drink

Multiple Choice

1.	4	6.	1	11.	3, 4
2.	1	7.	2	12.	1
3.	3	8.	2	13.	3
4.	2	9.	4	14.	2
5.	2	10.	2, 3, 1, 4	15.	4

Critical Thinking Exercise

1. The nurse should never leave a client who is potentially hemorrhaging. The nurse should use the call light to obtain assistance. She should assess the fundal characteristics. If the fundus is boggy, a circular massage is indicated.

2. If the client has clots in the vagina requiring evacuation, the LPN / LVN may be restricted in certain facilities. If an IV or IV medications are ordered, the LPN/LVN may not be able to perform these interventions.

3. Changes in vital signs indicative of blood loss–related problems include a drop in blood pressure and increased heart rate and respirations.

4. The client may initially be managed with uterine massage. If retained clots are evident, they will need to be evaluated. IV fluids may be given. If the blood loss is significant, blood products or volume expanders may be administered. Uterine atony may be managed with pharmacological intervention. Medications such as Pitocin and Methergine may be administered. If no measures are successful to manage the postpartum bleeding, surgical intervention may be indicated.

Chapter 11 Life Span Growth and Development

Matching

1.	C	6.	I
2.	D	7.	A
3.	E	8.	F
4.	J	9.	G
5.	B	10.	H

Fill in the Blanks

1. Tanner's Stages
2. Presbyopia, presbycusis
3. decline
4. Cataracts
5. hereditary
6. gender
7. symbolism
8. concrete operations
9. industry versus inferiority
10. peers

Multiple Choice

1.	4	6.	3	11.	1, 2, 3
2.	1	7.	2	12.	4
3.	2	8.	4	13.	2
4.	1, 2, 3	9.	2	14.	3
5.	3	10.	3	15.	2

Critical Thinking Exercise

1. According to Erikson, based on the child's age, he is in "Autonomy versus Shame and Doubt." According to Piaget, based on the child's age, he is in the "Preoperational."

2. To communicate and teach effectively to children and parents, the nurse needs to be aware of how a child thinks and understands and what physical issues are present in a child. This basic understanding will guide the nurse in their approach to many situations to produce a productive outcome. If one is not able to communicate on the "child's level," the nurse may not be able to accomplish the necessary tasks.

3. A child of this age should not be given a choice if none exists. Do not ask the child if he will get ready for the shot. Use of the word "shot" when first entering the room and having the syringe in sight may rapidly induce fear in the child of this age. Getting frustrated with the child would be inappropriate and less likely to occur if the nurse had knowledge of growth and development. Trying to take the child away from their support and comfort (the parent) will further impede the nurse's ability to accomplish this task. The nurse should avoid frightening discussions, speak at the child's eye level, and be specific about what the child is expected to do.

4. The father should be encouraged to be involved to participate as much as they are comfortable. Restraining the child for the injection may not be something each parent wants to do, but they can be helpful. The nurse needs to administer the injection, but a parent may help explain to the child what they need to do. Parents are the support and should be allowed to be present in the room at all times with this age of child. The parent should be encouraged to provide comfort after the injection.

Chapter 12 Illness Prevention, Health Promotion and Nutrition in Children

Matching

1. I
2. F
3. A
4. G
5. H

6. J
7. C
8. D
9. B
10. E

Fill in the Blanks

1. preschool
2. 5%
3. Fat
4. back seat
5. teething
6. iron
7. drowning, preschoolers
8. calcium
9. risk taking
10. toilet training

Multiple Choice

1.	3, 4	6.	2	11.	4
2.	3	7.	3	12.	4
3.	2, 3, 4	8.	4	13.	2
4.	1, 3, 4	9.	4	14.	1
5.	3	10.	2	15.	2

Critical Thinking Exercise

1. They learn to explore their environment by becoming more balanced and coordinated with walking. They learn to climb stairs, ride a tricycle. Toddlers may continue to put many objects into their mouth. They are learning to "mimic" adult behaviors by observing adults. They may start to play in or with water.

2. The independent nature of the toddler may put them at risk for injury. Gates need to be placed at the bottom and top of stairs. Rooms that are off limits for a child need to be blocked. Toddlers must be supervised at all times while outdoors playing, especially if near the road or water. Small objects must be kept away from toddlers. Small game pieces or coins may still be placed in the mouth and be a safety hazard. By "mimicking" adult behavior, the child may try to reach items in the kitchen or on the stove.

3. Parallel play is what is typical of this age of child. They enjoy playing next to but not actually with another child. They observe other children's behaviors, but are not able to play with another child at this stage.

4. Toilet training becomes a psychosocial issue during the toddler years. The child must physically be ready to begin or the process will not work. The child needs to be given positive feedback to encourage the behavior to continue.

5. Toddlers do not typically follow the three meals per day plan. They like to eat smaller amounts several times throughout the day. Parents need to understand that this is acceptable and provide nutritional offerings at multiple times. This will help keep the toddler matched with the energy and activity levels.

Chapter 13 Adapting Procedures in the Care of Children

Matching

1.	F	6.	B
2.	G	7.	C
3.	J	8.	D
4.	I	9.	H
5.	A	10.	F

Fill in the Blanks

1. retinas, lungs
2. fifth
3. pinna, ear, down

4. pressure
5. weight, kilograms, height, meters, squared
6. 36, months
7. equal, two, greater, two
8. age, size, condition, procedure
9. nares, pharynx, esophagus, stomach
10. tip, nose, tragus, ear, xiphoid, process

Multiple Choice

1.	1, 2, 4	6.	2	11.	4
2.	2	7.	2	12.	3
3.	4	8.	1	13.	3
4.	1, 2, 3	9.	3	14.	4
5.	3	10.	1, 2, 4	15.	2

Critical Thinking Exercise

1. With this tentative admitting diagnosis, the nurse would expect the testing to be ordered that would rule out many serious illnesses. These might include sepsis, appendicitis, pneumonia, or other respiratory or vial illnesses. The tests that would typically be done in a specific order include collecting urine before other painful testing is done, so that child would not become incontinent making urine collection more difficult, throat swabbing, blood testing with possible intravenous insertion at the same time, and lumbar puncture last.

2. With this age, the nurse should be honest with the child about what is going to be done to them. The parents should be encouraged to remain with the child as much as possible, but not be asked to assist in any restraining or collection of specimens if at all possible. The nurse will gain more cooperation by allowing the child to see some of the equipment being used, demonstrate on a doll or the parent and allow the child to possibly handle some of the equipment.

3. In a child of this age, the following vital signs would be able to appropriately be collected by the following methods:

    Temperature—Tympanic, remembering to pull the pinna of the ear up and back in a child that is over 3 years of age

    Pulse—Recommended to count apical pulse for 1 full minute

    Respiratory rate—Measure by auscultating lungs or by placing hand on abdomen, counting for 1 full minute

    Blood pressure—Manual or electric method using the upper arm as the preferred site

4. If a child is on a pediatric unit and further testing or procedures are indicated, the child should be taken out of the hospital room to a procedure or testing room. This will allow the child to have a "safe" place to return to with the parents. The parents should be allowed to remain with the child if at all possible. The nurse should be aware that the child may remember what was felt during the last time the test/procedure was performed, and cooperation may be more difficult to obtain. Extra time and attention may be needed.

Chapter 14 Care of the Hospitalized or Chronically Ill Child

Matching

1.	H	6.	G
2.	I	7.	A
3.	F	8.	B
4.	C	9.	E
5.	J	10.	D

Fill in the Blanks

1. deep breathing, incentive spirometer
2. lung expansion
3. conscious sedation
4. admission
5. Safe, secure
6. therapeutic play
7. hereditary condition
8. congenital condition
9. emotional
10. individualized education plan

Multiple Choice

1.	2	6.	4	11.	3
2.	1, 3, 4	7.	3	12.	1
3.	2	8.	4	13.	1
4.	3	9.	2	14.	2
5.	1, 2, 3, 4	10.	1, 2	15.	3

Critical Thinking Exercise

1. The 8-year-old child is at school-age level and is usually very industrious. They are interested in learning about their bodies and are able to understand basic concepts. By using a variety of methods to approach the teaching about the surgery, the new nurse should consider use of books written at a child's level, colored line drawings of the body parts involved, stuffed animals to show concepts through, or a basic DVD about surgery. Based on the child's questions and comfort level, the nurse can go into more detail.

2. The preoperative teaching needs include discussion and demonstration/ practice of coughing, deep breathing, turning in bed, splinting of an incision, use of incentive spirometer, discussion of pain rating tool and medication administration routes (including PCA pump), what will be expected regarding activity after surgery, dressing types, diet progression, and any specific questions the child or parents may have.

3. The postoperative needs include pain management, encouragement of activity when ordered, assessment of lung sounds and bowel sounds, pain level assessment and interventions (nonpharmacological and pharmacological) to

address pain, incision assessment and care, initiation of nutritional consumption, psychosocial needs (toys, movies, games, visits from family, including siblings if possible, and friends, if possible) and any other specific areas requiring more assessment.

4. Some unique ideas to implement the postoperative interventions include having the child blow bubbles or blow a pinwheel instead of a traditional incentive spirometer, providing fluids and food by fun cups and plates, making a game out of the activity, having child change a "dressing" on a doll or stuffed animal, providing a surgical mask for doll or stuffed animal and encouraging the child to draw pictures about the experience and how they are feeling to gain insight that they might not verbalize.

5. The parents need to be encouraged to be present and involved as much as they want to be. They know their child best and can be interpretive of non-verbal communication from the child. They will most likely be stressed and afraid for their child, so involving them in the care of their child will give them back a feeling of involvement and control of the situation.

Chapter 15 Care of the Child with Fluid, Electrolyte, and Acid-Base Disorders

Matching

1.	D	6.	A
2.	G	7.	E
3.	I	8.	B
4.	J	9.	C
5.	H	10.	F

Fill in the Blanks

1. 50%
2. 60%
3. 75%
4. Daily weight
5. Weight
6. gram, one
7. 10
8. percentage, weight
9. generalized, dependent
10. Hypervolemia

Multiple Choice

1.	3	6.	3	11.	2
2.	2	7.	2, 3, 4	12.	2
3.	3	8.	4	13.	4
4.	3	9.	2	14.	1, 2, 3
5.	2, 3	10.	3	15.	3

Critical Thinking Exercise

1. The nurse would need to focus on assessing for signs and symptoms of dehydration. In an infant, this would specifically include weight (without any clothing on), full set of vital signs, mucous membranes, skin turgor, urine output, presence of tears when crying, and anterior fontanel. If ordered by the physician, labs that might be assessed include urine specific gravity and ABGs. A weight loss calculation would be determined to identify the classification of dehydration. Another attempt would be made to assess the specific intake the child consumes and on what frequency. The child of this age should be receiving formula or breast milk with table foods.

2. The results of the assessment that would be anticipated in a child who is found to be dehydrated include rapid and thready pulse, low blood pressure, decreased urinary output, increased urine specific gravity, dry mucous membranes, absence of tears, inelastic skin turgor, and a sunken anterior fontanel.

3. Metabolic acidosis may occur in situations, including starvation, anorexia nervosa, bulimia, severe diarrhea, intestinal malabsorption, drug toxicity, diabetes, and renal failure.

4. Two potential nursing diagnoses might include "Decreased Fluid Volume Related to Deficient Fluid Intake" and "Imbalance Nutrition: Less than Body Requirements Related to Inadequate Nutritional Intake."

Chapter 16 Care of the Child with Neurologic and Sensory Disorders

Matching

1. I
2. G
3. H
4. J
5. B

6. A
7. C
8. D
9. F
10. E

Fill in the Blanks

1. 2
2. eustachian, tube, otitis, media
3. Tinnitus
4. Dyslexia
5. strabismus
6. hyperopia, myopia
7. trisomy, 21, chromosome
8. before, 5
9. Bacterial
10. cerebral, palsy

Multiple Choice

1.	3	6.	3	11.	2
2.	1, 3, 4	7.	3	12.	3
3.	2, 4	8.	4	13.	3
4.	2	9.	2	14.	4
5.	2, 3, 4	10.	4	15.	4

Critical Thinking Exercise

1. The medical term for ear infection is otitis media.
2. The younger child has the potential for more ear infections due to the shape of the eustachian tube. It is shorter and wider in the younger child. This allows bacteria to enter the middle ear more quickly and easily.
3. The signs and symptoms in an infant would include crying when drinking from a bottle or lying down, and pulling at the ear if an older infant. The verbal child would be able to complain of pain in the ear (otalgia). It is common for a child with an ear infection to also have an upper respiratory infection and fever. Irritability, vomiting, and diarrhea may also be present.
4. The treatment for recurrent otitis media is to have a myringotomy. A small plastic tube is inserted through the tympanic membrane to allow drainage from the middle ear. This will hopefully allow the antibiotics to eradicate the infection if the fluid is not constantly present.
5. Children who have myringotomy tubes in their ears need to take the following precautions: water should not be allowed into the ear. Bathing, showering, swimming, or other water activities should be carefully monitored. Earplugs should be worn during these times to prevent an infection from entering the middle ear.

Chapter 17 Care of the Child with Musculoskeletal Disorders

Matching

1.	F	6.	I
2.	A	7.	D
3.	J	8.	G
4.	E	9.	C
5.	H	10.	B

Fill in the Blanks

1. *Staphylococcus aureus*
2. distal femur, proximal tibia, proximal humerus
3. erythrocyte sedimentation rate
4. 10, 20
5. chemotherapy
6. independence
7. emotional

8. cervical spine
9. Severe scoliosis
10. growing pains

Multiple Choice

1.	3	6.	4	11.	2
2.	2, 3, 4	7.	1, 2, 3, 4	12.	1
3.	1	8.	3	13.	2, 3, 4
4.	3	9.	1	14.	2
5.	3	10.	2	15.	3

Critical Thinking Exercise

1. The child has emotional needs, such as safety and desire for diversional activities that are age appropriate, maintenance of daily routine and physical needs such as pain management, and frequent neurovascular assessments.
2. After a period of time in skeletal traction, the child will most likely have a hip-spica cast applied for continued healing with bone immobilization.
3. This situation requires further assessment into the cause of the injury. The possibility of abuse must be considered if there are other indicators such as behavior changes when the parents are present or the presence of bruises in various stages of healing.
4. One of the greatest challenges for the nurse caring for the child in traction would be to keep the child in proper alignment. The nursing diagnosis of: "Impaired Mobility Related to Musculoskeletal Impairment" would be appropriate.

Chapter 18 Care of the Child with Respiratory Disorders

Matching

1.	C	6.	A
2.	J	7.	D
3.	H	8.	B
4.	G	9.	E
5.	I	10.	F

Fill in the Blanks

1. sweat chloride test
2. Antibiotics
3. autosomal recessive
4. respiratory, gastrointestinal
5. Pneumothorax
6. smoke-free
7. status asthmaticus
8. SIDS, one, one

9. chest X-ray
10. Neonatal respiratory distress syndrome, premature

Multiple Choice

1.	3	6.	1	11.	4
2.	2, 3	7.	2	12.	1, 2, 3, 4
3.	2	8.	1, 3, 4	13.	3
4.	3	9.	2	14.	3
5.	2	10.	2	15.	2, 3, 4

Critical Thinking Exercise

1. Sudden infant death syndrome (SIDS) is the sudden, unexplained death of an infant under 1 year of age.
2. SIDS most often strikes infants between 2 and 4 months of age and is more common in males. It is the leading cause of death of infants between 1 month and 1 year of age.
3. In addition to being more prevalent in 2- to 4-month old males, other common factors in SIDS include Native American or African American descent, prematurity, low birth weight, multiple births, sleeping prone, maternal age less than 20 years, low socioeconomic status, exposure to passive smoke, and time of year. This 2-month-old male infant of Native American descent had numerous risk factors that predisposed him to SIDS, including being born prematurely and sleeping prone. Depending on the family's socioeconomic status, infant's birth weight, possibility of smoking in the home, this too, could have played yet another role in the infant's death.
4. The nurse has an important role in supporting the family. Providing knowledge can be used to help family members understand that the death was not their fault. Grandparents will need additional support from the nurse as well. They will be experiencing grief at the loss of their grandchild, but also extreme hurt to watch their own children suffer. The nurse should make sure that family members are allowed to hold the infant and receive handprint, footprints, and a lock of hair. The nurse should also provide the family with information about local support groups.
5. The main preventative measure is to place infants on their backs to sleep. The nurse plays an important role in educating the community about SIDS prevention whenever possible.

Chapter 19 Care of the Child with Cardiovascular Disorders

Matching

1.	G	6.	A
2.	H	7.	J
3.	F	8.	C
4.	I	9.	D
5.	B	10.	E

Fill in the Blanks

1. streptococcal
2. oxygen, fluid, electrolyte
3. aspirin
4. circumoral
5. erythrocyte sedimentation, Kawasaki
6. hyperlipidemia, fat, cholesterol
7. severe
8. transposition of the great arteries
9. narrowing, arch
10. no

Multiple Choice

1.	1, 2, 4	6.	4	11.	1, 2, 3
2.	1, 2, 3, 4	7.	2	12.	3
3.	3	8.	3	13.	2
4.	3	9.	2	14.	4
5.	2	10.	4	15.	4

Critical Thinking Exercise

1. Congestive heart failure (CHF) is the inability of the heart to pump enough blood throughout the body to maintain well-being. Blood can pool in the systemic venous circulation, which results in peripheral edema. CHF may be acute or chronic. The child will experience increasing dyspnea, or shortness of breath. Cardiac and respiratory rates increase. The circulatory deficits decrease cardiac output and can lead to cardiogenic shock. CHF can result from congenital or acquired heart defects.

2. The treatment of CHF targets the reduction of the workload of the heart to increase its efficiency.

3. Three common nursing diagnoses include Decreased Cardiac Output Related to Changes in Heart, Fluid Volume Excess Related to Inability of the Heart to Pump Effectively, and Ineffective Breathing Patterns Related to Excess Fluid Volume in Circulation and Lungs.

4. Five nursing interventions in the child with CHF include

   1. Weigh the child at the same time each day in the same clothing to detect subtle fluid and electrolyte changes.
   2. Take vital signs frequently, such as every 2–4 hours to detect any systemic changes.
   3. Monitor intake and output every 2 hours to detect and potential fluid volume shifts or issues.
   4. Assess heart and breath sounds every 2–4 hours to determine changes and presence of moist lung sounds.
   5. Encourage bed rest and a quiet environment to decrease workload on heart.

Chapter 20 Care of the Child with Hematologic or Lymphatic Disorders

Matching

1. C
2. E
3. D
4. B
5. F

6. G
7. J
8. I
9. A
10. H

Fill in the Blanks

1. straw
2. pain
3. hand washing
4. ill
5. iron
6. Thrombocytes

Multiple Choice

1. 2
2. 2
3. 3
4. 4
5. 2
6. 2

7. 1
8. 3
9. 1
10. 2
11. 4
12. 2

13. 3
14. 3
15. 2
16. 4
17. 2

Critical Thinking Exercise

1. Avoid those who are ill, keep immunizations current, keep him hydrated, and wash hands frequently.
2. The mother should call the physician if she believes her son is ill, has a temperature, is irritable or in pain, and/or is having shortness of breath.
3. The mother may give a warm bath, over-the-counter analgesics as prescribed by the pediatrician, massage, and distraction techniques.
4. Vaso-occlusive sickle cell crisis occurs when the sickle cells accumulate in a vessel and cause pain.

Chapter 21 Care of the Child with Immune Disorders

Matching

1. J
2. G
3. A
4. B
5. C

6. D
7. F
8. H
9. E
10. C

Fill in the Blanks

1. foreign
2. Candidiasis
3. OraQuick
4. JRA, SLE
5. history
6. natural immunity

Multiple Choice

1.	1	7.	3	13.	3
2.	3	8.	2	14.	1
3.	2	9.	3	15.	4
4.	4	10.	1	16.	2
5.	2	11.	2		
6.	4	12.	4		

Critical Thinking Exercise

1. A cesarean section.
2. The mother should feed her neonate formula.
3. She should practice protected sex, inform health care professionals of HIV status, avoid contaminating others with body fluids, and avoid breastfeeding infants.
4. The mother should take an antiretroviral agent.

Chapter 22 Care of the Child with Gastrointestinal Disorders

Matching

1.	F	6.	H
2.	G	7.	C
3.	I	8.	B
4.	A	9.	E
5.	J	10.	D

Fill in the Blanks

1. encouragement, support
2. ruptured appendix
3. irritation
4. kwashiorkor
5. **S**tabilize the child's condition, **I**dentify the toxic substance, **R**everse its effects, **E**liminate the substance from the child's body, and **S**upport the child (and parents) physically and psychologically.

6. Meckel's diverticulum
7. Hirschsprung's disease

Multiple Choice

1.	2	7.	2	13.	2
2.	2	8.	4	14.	4
3.	1	9.	2	15.	1
4.	3	10.	1	16.	3
5.	3	11.	1	17.	4
6.	4	12.	1	18.	1

Critical Thinking Exercise

1. Call for another health care professional to assess the client such as a nurse practitioner or physician, auscultate bowel sounds, assess level of consciousness and pulse oximetry, and obtain IV access.

2. Was the child exposed to any parasites while in Mexico, such as drinking water from the tap, around any animals, and what types of food did the client ingest? What intake has the client had in the last 24 to 48 hours? Has the client been able to keep liquids and solids down? Has the client ingested food or liquid and immediately experienced diarrhea? Has the client received his immunizations, and are they up-to-date?

3. Stool specimen; for occult blood, ova and parasite, culture and sensitivity. Serum labs: electrolytes, CBC, metabolic panel, and urinalysis.

4. Obtain IV access and infuse continuous IV fluids; transfer to a hospital if the client is stable.

Chapter 23 Care of the Child with Genitourinary Disorders

Matching

1.	D	6.	F
2.	C	7.	H
3.	B	8.	E
4.	A	9.	J
5.	I	10.	G

Fill in the Blanks

1. bed-wetting
2. Dysmenorrheal
3. Puberty
4. Hypospadias
5. Nephrolithiasis

Multiple Choice

1.	2	7.	4	13.	2
2.	3	8.	2	14.	3
3.	4	9.	1	15.	2
4.	2	10.	2	16.	3
5.	1	11.	3		
6.	2	12.	1		

Critical Thinking Exercise

1. Ecchymosis noted bilateral wrist and thigh areas.
2. You should report your findings to your supervisor so the child can be reviewed for possible sexual abuse.
3. Instruct the client on how to wipe the perineum from front to back whenever she urinates or has a bowel movement.
4. Offer foods and drinks that are nutritious and the client likes, offer movies and other activities that the client enjoys, allow the family to visit often and allow for independence whenever possible.

Chapter 24 Care of the Child with Integumentary Disorders

Matching

1.	I	6.	C
2.	D	7.	J
3.	F	8.	B
4.	E	9.	A
5.	G	10.	H

Fill in the Blanks

1. **A** = asymmetry of shape, **B** = border irregularity, **C** = color variation, **D** = diameter larger than 6mm, **E** = elevation of lesion
2. Dermatitis
3. Eczema
4. comedone
5. Cryotherapy
6. Melanin
7. thermal burns

Multiple Choice

1.	2	7.	4	13.	1
2.	3	8.	3	14.	3
3.	1	9.	1	15.	4
4.	2	10.	2	16.	2
5.	2	11.	3	17.	3
6.	3	12.	2		

Critical Thinking Exercise

1. Herpes simplex type 1 is a virus that causes oral lesions. The virus lays dormant until a trigger causes it to appear. This type of herpes is not sexually transmitted but can be transmitted on direct contact.
2. The virus lies dormant, and outbreaks can occur during times of emotional crisis, menses, fever, and exposure to extreme temperatures.
3. A medication, acyclovir (Zovirax), first applied to the area at the first signs of tingling helps to treat the lesion. Avoidance of triggers may prevent the lesion from appearing. If you suspect you are pregnant or become pregnant, it is important to inform your physician of this virus.
4. The lesion will become dry and heal in 8 to 10 days.

Chapter 25 Care of the Child with Endocrine Disorders

Matching

1.	E	6.	D
2.	J	7.	B
3.	H	8.	G
4.	I	9.	A
5.	F	10.	C

Fill in the Blanks

1. ADH
2. Exophthalmos
3. Insulin
4. feet
5. school
6. *Candida* vaginitis
7. two

Multiple Choice

1.	3	7.	3	13.	3
2.	4	8.	4	14.	2
3.	1	9.	2	15.	4
4.	3	10.	1	16.	3
5.	2	11.	3	17.	2
6.	1	12.	1		

Critical Thinking Exercise

1. Assess respiratory status and ensure proper airway.
2. Check blood glucose.

3. Normal saline
4. Potassium
5. Serum electrolytes

Chapter 26 Care of the Child with a Communicable Disease

Matching

1. D
2. F
3. H
4. J
5. I
6. A
7. C
8. G
9. B
10. E

Fill in the Blanks

1. Bioterrorism
2. Sexually transmitted infections (STI)
3. incubation
4. fomite
5. portal of entry

Multiple Choice

1. 2
2. 4
3. 2
4. 3
5. 1
6. 3
7. 1
8. 3
9. 4
10. 3
11. 4
12. 2
13. 3
14. 2
15. 2
16. 1
17. 2

Critical Thinking Exercise

1. How did the client obtain these marks? How long have they been there?
2. Cupping may cause these types of bruising.
3. Child abuse; does the explanation for the bruising correlate to the explanation provided by the parents?
4. How is the procedure performed? Does this procedure have the potential for causing other physical complications?
5. The nurse should respect the family's cultural beliefs in a nonjudgmental manner.

Chapter 27 Care of the Child with Psychosocial Disorders

Matching

1. F
2. E
3. G
4. A
5. C

6. J
7. B
8. I
9. H
10. D

Fill in the Blanks

1. suicidal ideation
2. *Diagnostic and Statistical Manual of Mental Disorders* (DSM-IV)
3. Asperger's
4. Tourette syndrome
5. child abuse
6. license
7. Bullying

Multiple Choice

1. 4
2. 2
3. 3
4. 1
5. 3
6. 3

7. 1
8. 3
9. 4
10. 4
11. 1
12. 2

13. 3
14. 2
15. 3
16. 1
17. 4
18. 2

Critical Thinking Exercise

1. Do you keep secrets from anyone in your home? Who told you to keep these secrets? Has anyone touched you down there (private or perineal area)?
2. Call the physician so bodily fluids can be obtained. Call your supervisor so the proper authorities may be notified.
3. You must notify the physician and your supervisor so the proper experts may become involved to deal with the emotional issues that arise.
4. A mental health professional who is trained to manage pediatric clients who suffer from abuse.

Chapter 28 Care of the Family with a Dying Child

Matching

1. G
2. H
3. I
4. J
5. A

6. C
7. E
8. B
9. D
10. F

Fill in the Blanks

1. time
2. needs
3. empathy
4. brain dead
5. loss, disbelief
6. temporary
7. brain injury

Multiple Choice

1. 2
2. 1
3. 3
4. 2
5. 4
6. 2

7. 3
8. 1
9. 3
10. 2
11. 4
12. 1

13. 3
14. 1
15. 3
16. 1

Critical Thinking Exercise

1. Review the medication administration record for times and amounts of medication given during the night shift. If medication was given via IV, ensure the IV site is patent. Discuss with the mother and the client their level of pain pre- and postmedication administration.
2. Ensure the client's current level of pain is manageable. If not, obtain pain medication and/or notify the physician regarding the client's pain management. Administer pain medication. Notify your supervisor so the parent's concerns can be addressed by administrative personnel.
3. Biofeedback, massage therapy, distraction, changing positions, application of heat and/or cold, application of menthol preparations, application of pressure and/or vibration.
4. Pain, alteration in management related to increased level of pain. Coping: family, compromised related to client's pain management regimen. Powerlessness, related to inability to promote comfort. Therapeutic regimen management, ineffective related to pain management.